when language runs dry

An Anthology for People with Chronic Pain and Their Allies

edited by
claire barrera & Meredith Butner

When Language Runs Dry

Mend My Dress Press
Tacoma, WA
MendMyDress.com

ISBN-13 978-0-9912354-4-5
Library of Congress Catalog-in-publication data available upon request

**Let a sufferer try to describe a pain in his
head to a doctor and language at once runs dry**

— Virginia Woolf, *On Being Ill*

table of contents

On Self Care • 139
Cover art • Corinne Teed

introduction

We've spent a lot of time in bed. We've had many meetings in bed, propped with pillows, laptops on the comforter. We've played card games together in bed when one or either or us couldn't get up to hang out otherwise. We've eaten meals in bed - meals for post-partum recovery, meals for an anti-inflammatory diet. We've talked on the phone or emailed from separate beds, tucked under the covers in the morning or at night. To make a zine about chronic pain, and then another, and then three more, we had to approach it in the ways our bodies and hearts asked us to. Sometimes it has been slow, or truncated, or uncomfortable. It has also been nourishing, connecting and validating.

Chronic pain can arise as the result of an injury, underlying illness, or without clear cause. Simply put, it is pain that continues when it should not, extending beyond the expected period of healing or in the absence of evidence of harm. It can be nagging or agonizing, episodic or incessant, mildly inconvenient or totally debilitating. Because it is a condition that is invisible, pain often goes without treatment or diagnosis. The chronic pain experience is not just physical, but also has serious emotional and social implications, intersecting with stress, depression, fatigue and anxiety in complex ways. Over the ten years we have worked on *When Language Runs Dry*, our own experiences of chronic pain and those of our contributors have fluctuated and morphed many times. To live with an illness that is about duration and invisibility is to experience an incredible gamut of feeling, emotion and understanding.

Pain is often described as unspeakable, a sensation so consuming that it can dismantle language. Words fail in the face of overwhelming distress: we fall on the floor, we cry, we moan, we scream. Pain dulls other senses, pulls attention inward. Pain can make us fuzzy, inarticulate; isolated inside an experience that we cannot easily communicate. Pain begs us to withdraw, we may no longer participate in our communities the way we once could. In this way, pain can upend a personal sense of identity. When a person is no longer able to define themselves, their world, and their beliefs as they once did, an empty space remains. A lack of education and understanding in the larger culture can deepen this sense of speechlessness.

When we first conceived of this zine it came from real, dire need for stories and connection. Both of us were in the throes of severe flare-ups. Our daily work was getting through pain moment to moment, and navigating all the systems of care and bureaucracies that come with illness. Our other selves had fallen away in subservience to survival. *When Language Runs Dry* quickly became a piece of that survival. Chronically ill and disabled folks need to speak, to be seen and to be supported as a matter of life or death. We also need to build community with each other and solidarity with our allies. For both of us, this zine was the only creative project we were able to engage in for years. Often it was one of the few social activities available to us. In this way it was a lifeline. It paved the way for us to find new ways of being in the world and eventually reconnect with other aspects of ourselves.

When Language Runs Dry has attempted to fill in the silence where stories of those with chronic pain should be. We could never have done so alone. We are privileged to represent so many perspectives within these pages. From the acute moments of crisis, when sense of self and community is shattered, to periods of maintenance where new identities, meaning and self-care practices are forged, *When Language Runs Dry* has created a platform for the diversity of voices we all need to hear. People with chronic pain have a lot to teach the larger community about bodies, care and support, trauma, culture and identity - all of these topics and many more have been covered by our incredible contributors through poetry, essays and comics. This anthology is for everyone. We hope it continues to add dimension to the narrative of life with chronic pain and offers readers inspiration to find language to share their own experiences.

Take care,

claire & Meredith

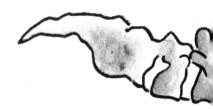

on illness and injury

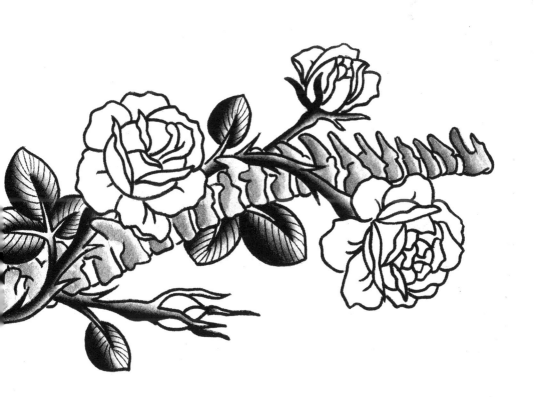

McGill - Melzack Pain Questionnaire

Patient's Name_____ Date_____ Time_____ am/pm
Analgesic(s)_____ Dosage_____ Time Given_____ am/pm
_____ Dosage_____ Time Given_____ am/pm

Analgesic Time Difference (hours): +4 +1 +2 +3
PRI: S_____ A_____ E_____ M(S)_____ M(AE)_____ M(T)_____ PRI'T)_____
     (1-10)   (11-15) (16)   (17-19)   (20)   (17-20)   (1-20)

1 FLICKERING ___	11 TIRING ___
QUIVERING ___	EXHAUSTING ___
PULSING ___	12 SICKENING ___
THROBBING ___	SUFFOCATING ___
BEATING ___	13 FEARFUL ___
POUNDING ___	FRIGHTFUL ___
2 JUMPING ___	TERRIFYING ___
FLASHING ___	14 PUNISHING ___
SHOOTING ___	GRUELLING ___
3 PRICKING ___	CRUEL ___
BORING ___	VICIOUS ___
DRILLING ___	KILLING ___
STABBING ___	15 WRETCHED ___
LANCINATING ___	BLINDING ___
4 SHARP ___	16 ANNOYING ___
CUTTING ___	TROUBLESOME ___
LACERATING ___	MISERABLE ___
5 PINCHING ___	INTENSE ___
PRESSING ___	UNBEARABLE ___
GNAWING ___	17 SPREADING ___
CRAMPING ___	RADIATING ___
CRUSHING ___	PENETRATING ___
6 TUGGING ___	PIERCING ___
PULLING ___	18 TIGHT ___
WRENCHING ___	NUMB ___
7 HOT ___	DRAWING ___
BURNING ___	SQUEEZING ___
SCALDING ___	TEARING ___
SEARING ___	19 COOL ___
8 TINGLING ___	COLD ___
ITCHY ___	FREEZING ___
SMARTING ___	20 NAGGING ___
STINGING ___	NAUSEATING ___
9 DULL ___	AGONIZING ___
SORE ___	DREADFUL ___
HURTING ___	TORTURING ___
ACHING ___	PPI
HEAVY ___	0 No pain ___
10 TENDER ___	1 MILD ___
TAUT ___	2 DISCOMFORTING ___
RASPING ___	3 DISTRESSING ___
SPLITTING ___	4 HORRIBLE ___
	5 EXCRUCIATING ___

PPI_____ COMMENTS:

CONSTANT ___
PERIODIC ___
BRIEF ___

ACCOMPANYING SYMPTOMS:	SLEEP:	FOOD INTAKE:
NAUSEA ___	GOOD ___	GOOD ___
HEADACHE ___	FITFUL ___	SOME ___
DIZZINESS ___	CAN'T SLEEP ___	LITTLE ___
DROWSINESS ___	COMMENTS:	NONE ___
CONSTIPATION ___		COMMENTS:
DIARRHEA ___		
COMMENTS:	ACTIVITY:	COMMENTS:
	GOOD ___	
	SOME ___	
	LITTLE ___	
	NONE ___	

Emily Klamer

understanding pain

The way I understood pain then:

- Most of the pain I dealt with before the onset of my degenerative disc disease (DDD) was sharply external in origin: bike accidents, rollerblade adventures gone awry, second degree burns from car wrecks, etc. In these instances, there was a direct cause of my pain: unexpected impact with concrete and wrought iron, rapidly deployed airbags, sharp metal slicing my skin.

- Pain was usually a result of an unexpected accident, some horrible misfortune that had announced itself, uninvited. But I always knew that the pain was temporary, there was relief in the knowledge that all pain would eventually fade. Pain didn't keep me up at night.

- Because pain was usually doled out by foreign objects, there were certain measures I could take in order to lessen or minimize injury: helmets, knee and elbow pads, seatbelts, common sense, caution.

- Pain was the result of visible wounds that could be seen and treated accordingly. A band-aid and Neosporin usually did the trick, and if not, stitches were the more hardcore and slightly glamorous alternative.

- The visibility of the wounds made asking for help simple or even unnecessary. The wound itself communicated its needs to be closed up, treated, and healed. Blood was the quintessential "red flag" that something was indeed wrong. Blood and pus tend to speak for themselves!

- When I was younger, I took for granted my body's capacity to heal. I never thought that those cuts, burns, or scrapes would gape open or ooze forever. I knew that at some point, the bleeding would stop, the scabs would form and eventually be sloughed off by time. Even resulting scar tissue was evidence that my body was resilient and strong.

- The tangibility of my pain was validating: it was something that could be seen, named, touched. It was a known pathology, something easily diagnosed and treated. I never doubted the sincerity of my pain or the fact that wounds and their consequent pain needed to be dealt with or that I deserved care.

- Pain could be romanticized, and I remember even fantasizing about being in great pain so that my loved ones may lament over my plight and fulfill my every desire. Of course, this was before the onset of my very own chronic pain, which shattered the illusion that the existence of pain guaranteed a cushy yet tragic life.

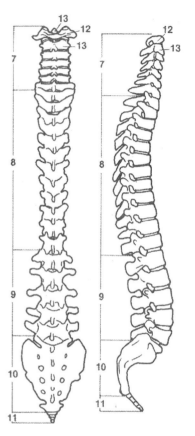

The way I understand pain now:

- With the diagnosis and onset of degenerative disc disease (a condition in which the jelly-like core of the discs in between the vertebrae degenerate, causing nerve disruption), the way that I conceptualize pain has been shifted: no longer an external offense, this pain is resonating from inside. People disagree about the cause of DDD, which leaves many of us diagnosed with it in an uncomfortably ambiguous space. While disc degeneration does not necessitate pain and is even normal as we age, I was diagnosed with it when I was 19 years old and have constant, low to mid grade pain, a combination that is kind of rare.

- I have been experiencing chronic pain for a couple years now, which doesn't really bode well. In the beginning, it was hard for me to just get past the label, 'degenerative disc disease,' which has a certain ring of doom-and-gloom to it. Chronic pain, in my experience, has certainly caused feelings of despair and hopelessness, which are equally as immobilizing as the pain itself.

- In the case of chronic pain resulting from DDD, there was nothing (as far as I know) I could have done in order to stop it. In some ways, this inevitability makes living with this condition almost easier for me, as it makes pain more of a fact of life than something I could have prevented.

- The source of constant back pain is invisible, at least to the naked eye. This makes both the identification and treatment of the pain uncertain, especially without the use of hi-tech medical equipment like x-rays and MRIs.

- My close ones usually don't know I am in pain unless I tell them or they can read my body language. Because I don't even know the "right way" to treat my back pain, it's hard to ask my friends for help. Chronic pain also lacks the urgency acute pain possesses, which redefines the parameters of treatment into a more long-term process. At this point, I am still dependent on doctors, as I do not yet have friends that are chiropractors, orthopedic surgeons, or miracle workers.

- In the case of DDD, there isn't a wound to heal. I can only slow the process of the degeneration and mitigate its effects with therapy, adjustments, and drugs (a trio that necessitates health insurance, which is another story).

- Because my back pain isn't tangible (I even have a hard time describing where exactly the pain is or what it feels like), I sometimes struggle with feelings that the pain is less real or less legitimate than acute pain. This also affects how and when I ask for help (see above).

- There's nothing like a diagnosis of potential life long pain to deflate the tragic romanticization of bodily trauma. Living with chronic pain has definitely caused me to redefine and expand the meaning of pain. I identify this pain as mine; it has become part of my identity, like every other life altering experience.

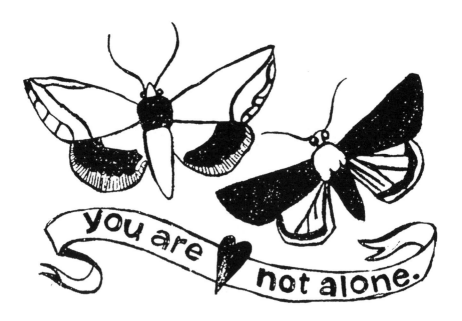

Noemi Martinez

because we do not fit, we are a threat

Today I hate my legs. The feeling of cotton, fuzzy numb almost pain but not quite.

Quick fix of provoked pain-hey they are still alive.

Today I hate my fingertips. Numb, almost frost bitten sensation. I look at them and say I hate you.

Pain is the way of life, Gloria Anzaldua

Although all your cultures reject the idea that you can know the other, you believe that besides love, pain might open this closed passage by reaching through the wound to connect. Wounds cause you to shift consciousness-they either open you to the greater reality normally blocked by your habitual point of you or else shut you down. Using wounds as openings to become vulnerable and available (present) to others means staying in your body - Gloria in This Bridge We Call home: Radical Visions of Transformation.

But really Gloria, really? The only thing pain does is make you present, reminds you that you are IN your body.

Staying in a body in pain and using wounds as opening to others-to trigger compassion-defies all conventional wisdom. - Suzanne Bost, writing in "Gloria Anzaldua's Mestiza Pain" *Aztlan Journal*, 30:2, Fall 2005.

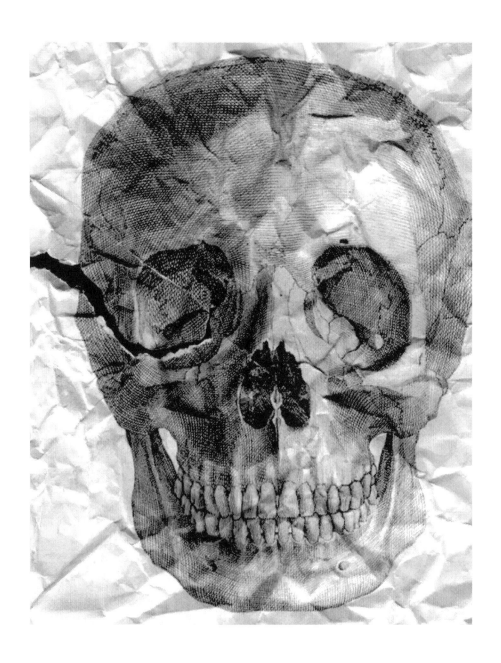

reconstruction
a collage of experiential components sifting through and choosing what to build a new life on

"Most individuals who have sustained more than a mild
traumatic brain injury neither die nor fully recover."

Understanding what happened to me took time

Bifrontal bitemporal hemorrhagic contusions edema increased
density of interhemispheric fissure of frontal lobes tentorial
acute subdural hematoma subarachnoid hemorrhage right
temporal bone longitudinal fracture temporoparietal extra
cranial soft tissue

I lost a week of memory, and chunks of time
dropped out of the weeks following.
The last thing I remember was getting on my bicycle
at 5:30 am to go to work on a Saturday morning,
though I question that as a
memory since it was a routine action.

Next I remember puking on myself,
pissing myself and pulling out my last IV

Opacification of the frontal sinuses ethmoid sinuses and multiple
right mastoid air cells largest confluent hematoma within the
inferior lateral left frontal lobe anterior cranial fossa contrecoup
injury convexity grossly stable

Once my continuous memory was re-engaged,
I digested my situation in small bits

"You were hit by a car." "It was hit and run." "The cops found
your body at the intersection." "You've been in the hospital for a
few days."

Skull fracture, intracranial hemorrhaging, multiple cerebral contusions, damaged ear canal and ear drum.

Stories filled in the blanks

"You argued that you didn't need intubation until you finally ripped out the lung tube yourself, earning you the nickname 'Houdini' in ICU because no one could understand how you removed the tube while in the restraints mandated by heavy sedation."

Despite the subsequent necessity
for vocal chord surgery months later,
this story provided me the image of myself as a fighter
that I appreciated.

"The Emergency Department staff commented on the strength and volume of your scream during your seizure."

Two nurses applauded the first time they saw me
walk down the hall in the Brain Recovery Unit
without using the wall as a guide.
At discharge I was aware of the biggest challenges:
Accepting recovery as a long-term process
Accepting the uncertain outcomes of recovery

I left the hospital with a kind of pain I had never experienced
before, and, armed with a very basic understanding,
started the process of re-entering my life and the world.
Writing became an important tool.

So here now is writing and expression post-cranial impact,
partly motivated by a desire for cognitive exercise,
most urgently motivated by a need for an outlet.
The desperation not being felt every moment of everyday,
but when there, being felt so absolutely. On the worst days,
writing is not a possibility since pain can render the smallest of
movements unbearably difficult.

"Don't go outside by yourself for the first week after discharge."

I didn't take the doctor's precaution seriously
until I attempted to navigate a New York City sidewalk as a
brain-injured person. All senses affected, over-sensitive,

under-sensitive,in a post-trauma body and mind
Someone five feet away feels dangerously close
I HAVE A BROKEN HEAD. PLEASE DON'T BUMP INTO ME.
PLEASE GIVE ME SOME SPACE.
Minimal filter for screening stimuli
leading to being overwhelmed quicklyDISTRACTED
Focus taking such energy
Every intersection a potential hazard,
every person passing an obstacle
The right sound at the right moment triggers adrenaline
An almost-slip on ice feels like dying
Slowing time to thread-bare
Squeezing through to the other side

CAR TIRES ON STREET, talking, SIRENS, laughing, BANG!!!
All SO close
This will pass. This will fade. Wait it out.

A high school kid's prank of jumping and screaming in my face

"WELCOME TO STANTON AND ELDRIDGE!!!!!!!!!!!!!!!"

This will pass. This will fade. Wait it out.

"What have you been up to lately?"

A lot of time at home
Time in my head, not always so helpful
Crying
MAD!!!
thankful to be alive
MAD!!!
Crying
Crying
ANGRY
I am lucky to be alive
Why the fuck is this happening to me?
Why am I not supporting myself by now?
I am not utilizing my time well
I should be doing _____.
Etc. (repeat X 100)

One part of me recognizes that I am walking, talking and
connected with my personality and uses it as a justification
for being hard on myself: I should be back to my previous life
routines, why am I not back to supporting myself?
Another part of me recognizes that I CONSTANTLY feel
DIFFERENT. My filter for receiving my experience has changed,
and I walk around, best case: feeling like cotton wrapped around
my head, float-walking; worst case: out-of-body, in pain,
angry at everyone, sad at every word exchanged.

Time at home also afforded me the opportunity
for self-education in medical terminology laden manuscripts
and experiential narratives (not much between) and the
satisfaction at finding that so many details of my experience
are common to survivors of TBI.
Learning how to speak about my experience
To speak a new language
Retrograde amnesia, amnestic disorder, hypervigilance, ocular
fatigue, cognitive fatigue, provoked vertigo, visual-vestibular
disturbances, anosmia
To attack the piles of papers
Medical funding applications
To become an advocate for myself in continuing recovery

The smells
In the beginning I said, "I still have no sense of smell,
but sometimes I get these smells stuck in there."
I received absolutely no response
I learned, on my own, of the common experience of
OLFACTORY HALLUCINATIONS
and later understood, on my own,
that I might be having temporal lobe seizures
Only when I used the newly acquired vocabulary with
health care providers were they able to address
this possible issue
"How long have you been experiencing them?"
Pretty much since discharge.
"How often do you have them?"
Multiple times a day.
"We need to get you on Keppra."

Outpatient recovery: Trauma Rehabilitation Occupational
Therapy
Physical Therapy Ear, Nose and Throat Neurology
Neuropsychology

The brain is a tricky, intricate thing. Monitoring progress
is the primary method for deciphering how a person
might present their brain damage. My husband, Ethan
learned this early on when he asked a neurologist
what issues I might struggle with given the evident
brain damage.

"We could speculate on the problems that may manifest by
looking at the CT, but we don't. We discern issues for a person in
recovery as they are encountered."

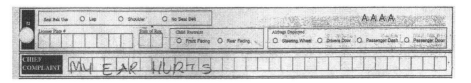

The most illustrative example of the tool of evaluation:
Roughly 15 hours of neuropsychological evaluations
compiled into a 12 page assessment
My life
My new cognitive, psychological and emotional functioning and
capabilities
In 12 pages

"Most notable are Ms. Anderson's executive functioning deficits,
reduced visual scanning abilities and problems with attentional
controls. Cognitive Disorder Not Otherwise Specified
DSM-IV 294.9"

I am being assessed

"Has anyone told you that you have done or said sexually
inappropriate things since acquiring a TBI?"

I am being assessed
This will pass. This will fade. Wait it out.
This feeling of being judged spilled into all parts of my life
Having to overcome misperceptions of brain injuries

by aggressively pursuing getting back to work
Feeling that I had to prove myself
Fearing the gazes of friends and acquaintances
Feeling they were searching my countenance for signs of change

I am okay.
I am okay.
"What are you doing today, Heather?"
Well, I just walked to and from the hospital for appointments
that took hours
and that is all my body currently can handle in one day
This is what I have to offer?

Wanting everyone to know I am okay.
Not wanting to ask for help
I am okay.
Angry when I don't get the help I am not asking for

Mom, Dad, Brothers:
Where were you?
Why didn't you come out to see me when I could've died?
Mom and Dad,
I know you have no money.
Adrian,
I know you are supporting Mom right now.
Travis,
I know you just got out of prison.
But why didn't any of you come to see me?
It's okay.
I am okay.

Learning that my social outlets are different now.
No, I can't meet you guys at the bar tonight.
No, I can't handle going to a show yet.
Which restaurant? Is it loud there?
How late do you want to meet?

Wanting to believe I am okay
.

Learning how to talk to specific individuals about it

"Are you feeling better?"

Yeah, I got a couple good night's sleep and feel better.
"See? It was all in your head!"

Trying to communicate the spectrum of pain
that I am now familiar with in a way that
will make sense to people
"How are you?"
(internal answer:
After the initial continuous axe-in-the-head pain that lasted
the first two months, my pain branched out into a family
each member with its own personality, each with its own
visitation schedule
There is the pain of headaches that last 2-4 days
tight, sometimes sharp-edged pain
severe enough to make life routines those days difficult
There is the pain that shoots or cuts through
pulsing anywhere from a few seconds to half an hour
an undeniable interruption
once, twice, or multiple times a day
There is the pain that feels like pressure, a squeeze in one area of
my brain
hitching a ride for a day here and there
There is the pain of radiating discomfort
usually specific to the right side of my head
which makes me feel unsafe sleeping on the right side of my head
like it is still tender and I may crush it by lying on it)
The answer I projected:
I have a brain-injury headache today.

"You know what cures that?"
(Squirts water in my eye with a spray bottle)

Trying to communicate that this isn't something that goes away

"Are things better?"
I don't know what my life will be like in
6 months, 1 year, or 2 years.
There is no 'better'. There is just me.

The Question
Customers at the café I work at somehow knew my entire story
Health care providers attempt to facilitate a discussion for

future risk reduction
"Were you wearing a helmet?"
An insulting, unnecessary, and sometimes inadvertent
implication of responsibility
I HAVE GLEANED ALL THE MEANING POSSIBLE
FROM THIS EXPERIENCE

Friends and family playing tough love
"You gonna wear a helmet now, Heather?"
I don't even know when I can get back on a bicycle

Dr.: "I don't think you should ride a bicycle on the streets of New
York City again."

Few people who ask if I was wearing a helmet
ask about the person who was driving the car
that hit me and left me in the street,
not knowing if I died
Never to know if I lived or died

1st and 4th
I walk past the intersection a lot
on my walk to the hospital
on my way to work
I notice it every time
"You need to find the meaning in this experience."
"This incident is a sign. You need to listen to what the universe is
trying to tell you."

I think of it every fucking time
This will pass. This will fade. Wait it out.

"In considering community re-entry as an outcome measure, we
are left with the problem of deciding which community we are
considering."

I am working on incorporating this experience
into who I am. It has helped to connect with people
who have had similar experiences, finding
inspiration and power through knowledge sharing.
Experiencing a reinforced alliance with my mother
who has dealt with Rheumatoid Arthritis for almost
20 years now.

Accepting that I am changed.
"Transitioning into new limitations."

I had a conversation with a woman who is a few years out from
her brain injury recently. I was shocked when she revealed
that she carries with her at all times a picture of herself in the
hospital, in a coma, soon after the trauma that caused her brain
injury. I twisted inside my head trying to understand. Another
woman said, "It's a birth picture."
And it clicked.
In my mind, I have allied her empowerment
through carrying that photograph with an action
that I engaged in shortly after discharge.
I took the pair of pants that the EMTs cut off my body
and I mended them
Seams, straight up the front
And I wear them sometimes
Wearing my trauma out in the open, up front
seams invisible to most, except me
Most importantly
I keep them
A concretization of my desire to piece things back together
A beginning of empowering myself through this experience

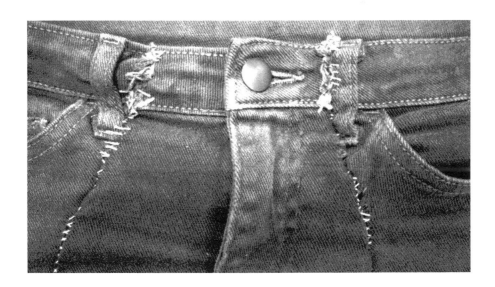

Some has passed. Some will not fade. No more waiting.

"I am still me, just MORE."

I hang onto this as I enter a new time of uncertainty:
The realization that I may be having seizures,
the efforts to find a definitive answer,
the re-acceptance that the recovery process is one
NOT of waiting
but LIVING

Of re-learning how to live my life
Of getting to know the person I am now

Fragments, flashes of memory that I don't recognize
Familiar but unrecognizable
Like pieces of myself that I don't know yet
I smile, excited by prospects,
Not knowing if it's a piece I just never noticed before
Or if it's something yet to come

I am a new person.

SICK

A Visual Account of an Invisible Disability

by Annie Murphy

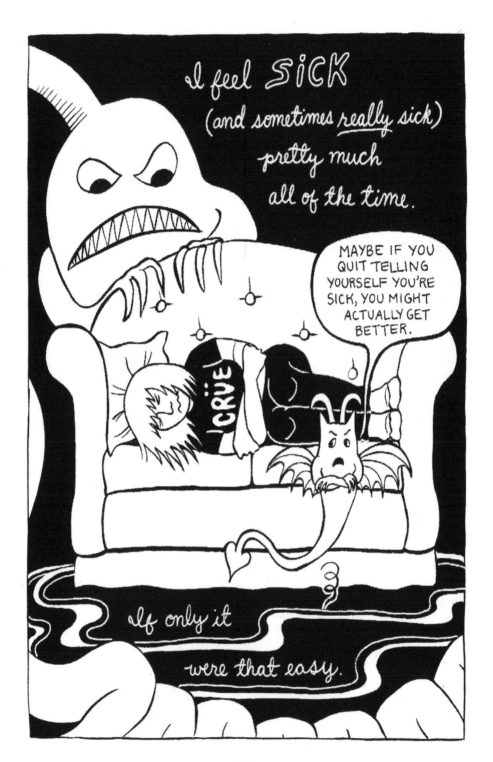

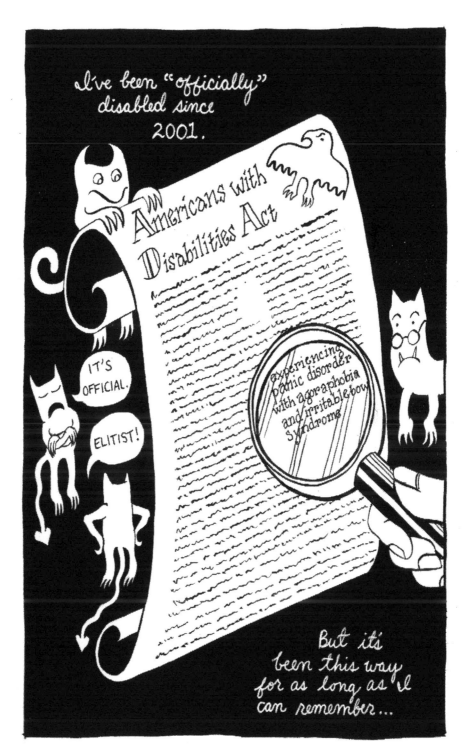

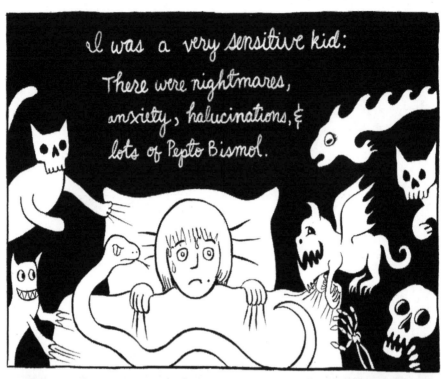

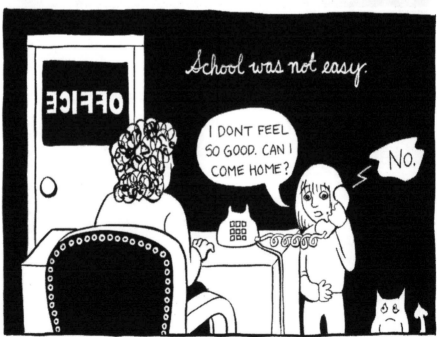

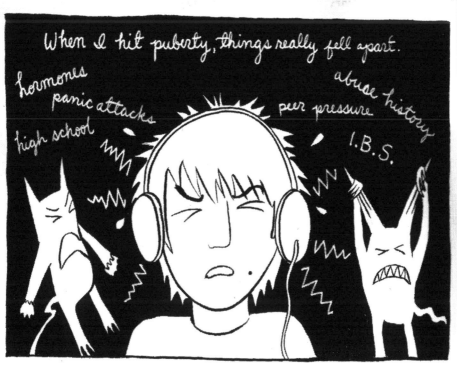

When I hit puberty, things really fell apart.

hormones
panic attacks
high school
peer pressure
abuse history
I.B.S.

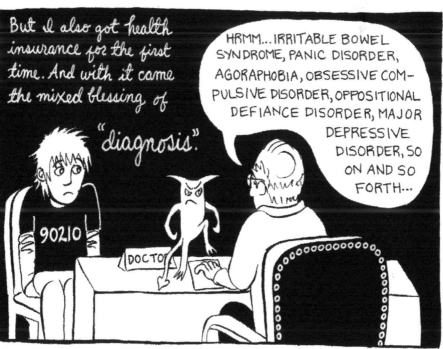

But I also got health insurance for the first time. And with it came the mixed blessing of "diagnosis."

90210

DOCTOR

HRMM... IRRITABLE BOWEL SYNDROME, PANIC DISORDER, AGORAPHOBIA, OBSESSIVE COMPULSIVE DISORDER, OPPOSITIONAL DEFIANCE DISORDER, MAJOR DEPRESSIVE DISORDER, SO ON AND SO FORTH...

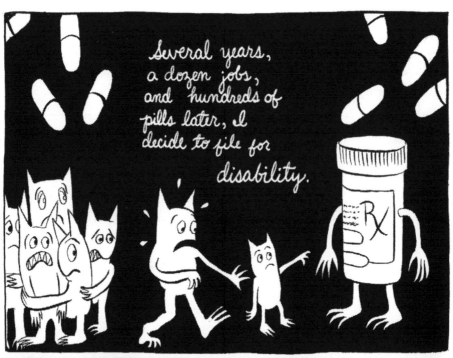

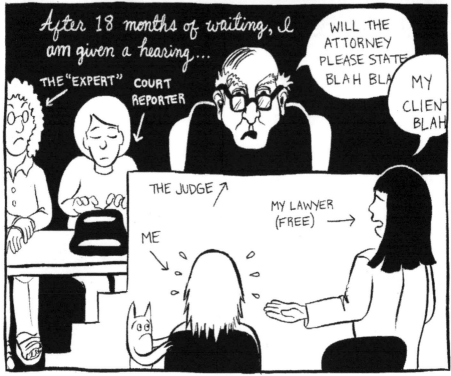

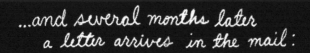

...and several months later
a letter arrives in the mail:

Social Security Administration
Portland, OR

Congratulations,
you are
officially

DISABLED

but
we will be checking up on
you periodically just to make
sure you are still disabled and
we may hire a private investigator to
track you, so no gainful employment, etc. blah, blah

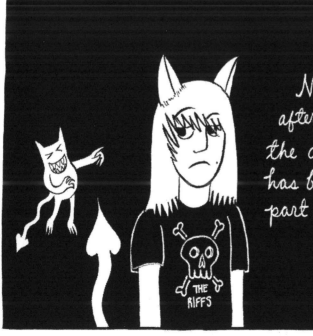

THE
RIFFS

Now,
after 8 years,
the disability
has become a
part of me.

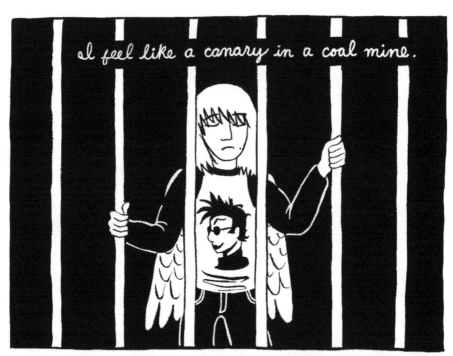

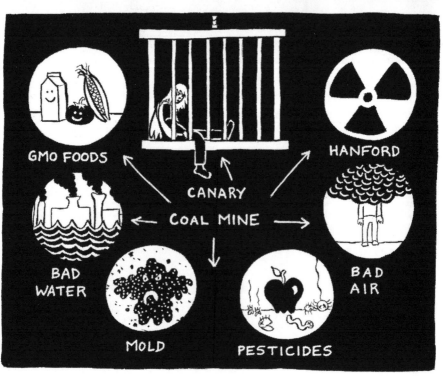

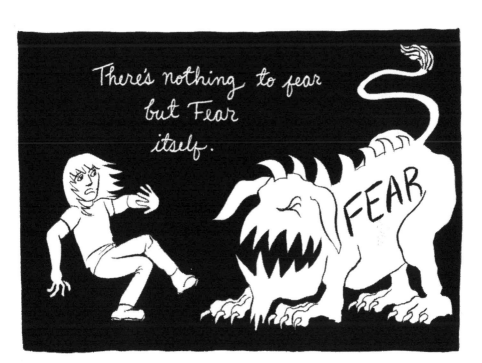

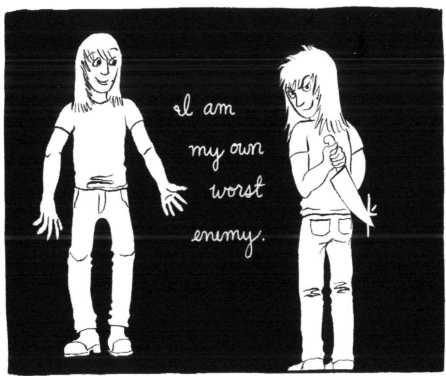

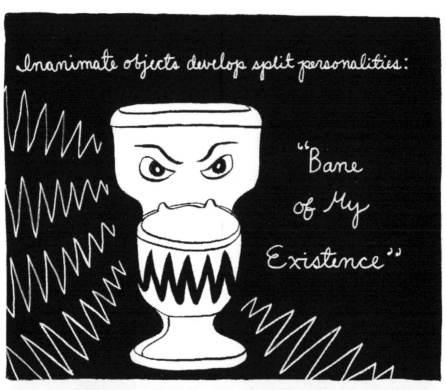

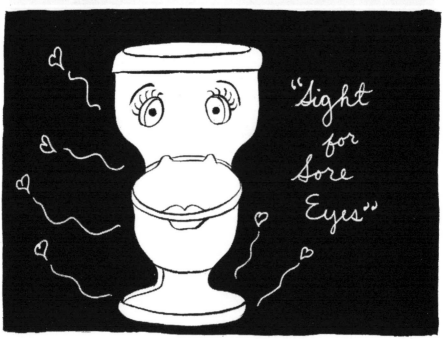

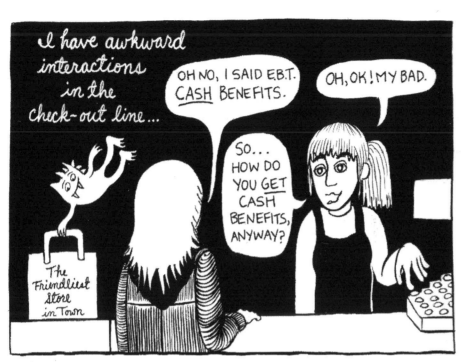

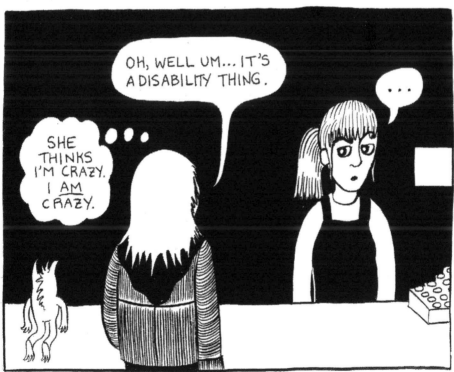

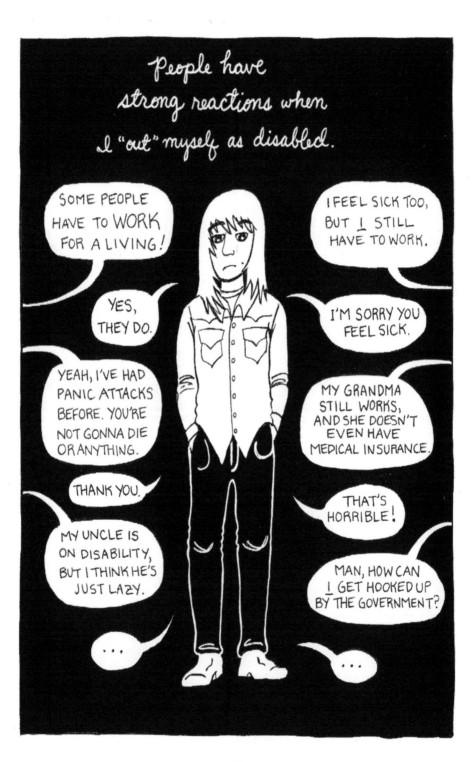

It can be pretty hard to field all the questions and comments, even from the well-meaners (those who want to help me get better, a.k.a. "fix" me).

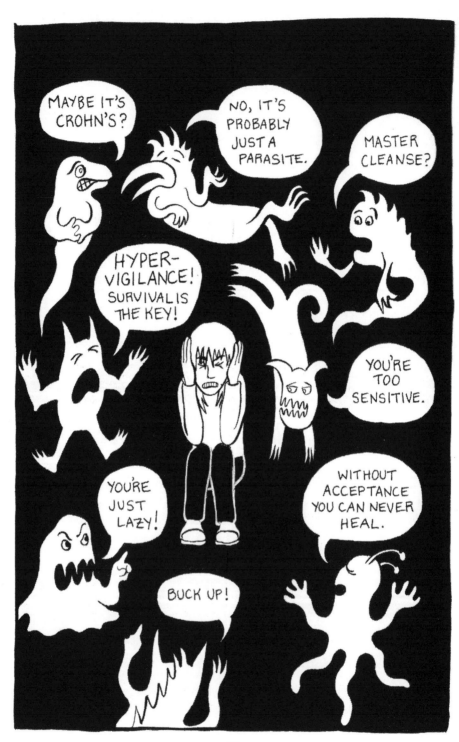

40

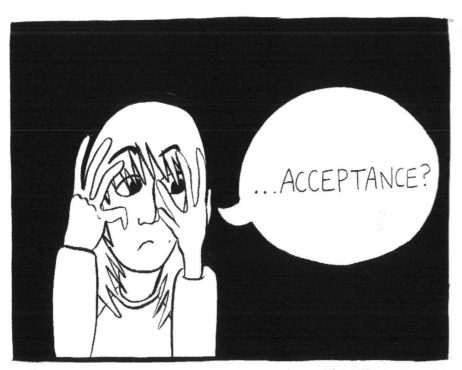

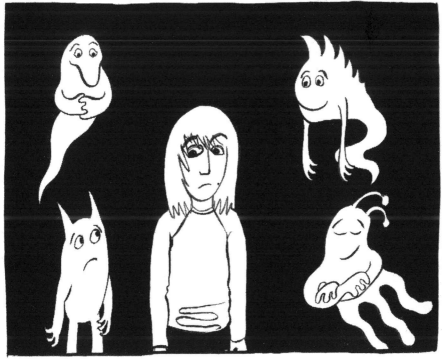

41

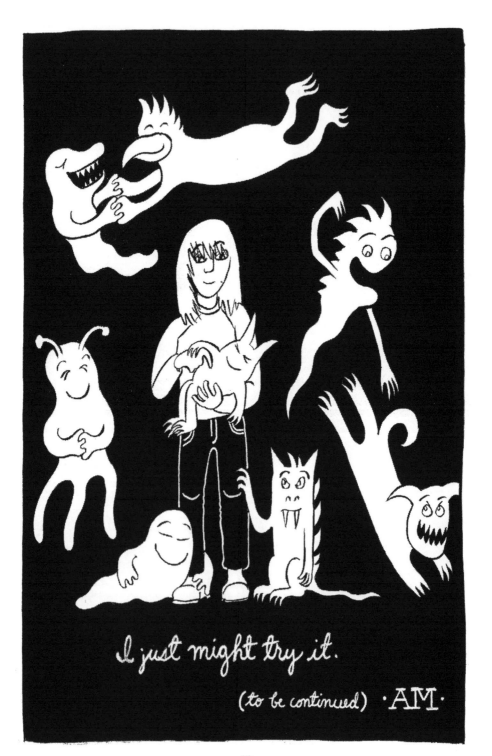

I just might try it.

(to be continued) ·AM·

anterior discectomy

While I was asleep, they slit my throat.
With that said, there is nothing for me to say about sex
Except to say, that after
When she fucked me
I could not understand what was happening
Which is not to say that I did not want her to
I did
More than anything
But not for the pleasure of it
But instead for the obliteration of death
For the obliteration of this, the failing of my flesh
That my body broke
Now and forever
Never the same
The hidden scar, a tender slit across tender flesh
And deep inside the break spreads away from the pulled
apart place
And so I wanted her to fuck me, to fuck the tender slit in
tender flesh
But not because I loved her, and not because I loved it,
I do
More than anything
But instead, because we are going to die
This body, this flesh, all that I have, no more to come,
Because that slit pierced me through, pulled me open
Like the dream of her hands prying me apart
Liquid wet lava pouring out
And nothing left, save the sea

on bravery

> *"Know that whatever it is you have been doing to survive deserves recognition and honoring, even if you don't particularly like it or if it's not serving you well anymore. Know that if you are alive right now you have been practicing self-defense. You have pathways in your psyche that have kept you in some ways safe, and they deserve thanks. Also, it is hard to change all at once, so take what you can from how you've been surviving so far, put it in your pocket for reference." -Doris Zine #25*

Pain crept into my life so slowly I didn't even need to make room for it. Introducing itself with a tug it felt, at first, like nothing more than a pulled muscle in my right leg. Now, as I trace injury back through eight years of journals, I see that it wasn't until a couple of months later that I started to make anything of the increasing discomfort I was feeling in my back and leg and sought out the help of a doctor.

Back then, I defined myself by the things that I made: my projects, music, and art. I was working a full time job, playing in bands, and running a show and recording space with friends. I had started sewing and getting involved in crafts and organizing. I felt I existed in what I brought to my community.

When pain demanded space and attention I resisted accommodating it. Sure, I gave injury some of my time by keeping therapy and doctor appointments, but I never slowed down the way I needed to and I refused to let it stop me. I felt more protective of my projects than my body and fought against the pain that was making me unproductive. I ignored the discomfort when I could, pressed on with what I felt I needed to get done and rested in tears and privacy at the end of the day. I told myself I was doing what I needed to do - I was being brave.

I grew up in a sunny Southern California suburb, the middle child to a middle class family. While illness and injury were never a big part of my childhood I learned early on that, in my family at least, being sick usually meant giving something up. My parents made it clear that if my siblings or I were too sick to go to school then we were too sick to play or participate in after school activities that day as well. In my elementary and middle school years I was devoted to dance and children's theater and would weigh every sore throat or sniffle against missing rehearsal or time in the neighborhood with friends.

If I ever did give in to sickness it usually meant I was actually really ill, resulting in a highly despised visit to the doctor and a round of antibiotics for bronchitis, strep throat, or whatever it was that had grabbed onto me. Strangely, my love for performance has always been coupled with contradictory feelings of hatred for being the center of attention. Detesting how invasive attention can feel, being *examined* by a doctor was an agony I would choose to avoid if at all possible.

I remember some days, in the time between school and dinner, when after getting us settled into our homework or tv programs my mom would tell my siblings and I she was *going to go lay down for a bit*. I knew then that Excedrin was her preferred brand of headache medicine and she always kept a few of those chalky white pills in a little tin in her purse. It wasn't until I started having migraine headaches of my own that I was even aware of the name for the kind of pain she was regularly bearing. She never made it known, never complained, never let her pain come between her and her family.

Though there was a lot of love in our home, comfort seemed to sometimes fail us. I would think hard before ever calling out to my parents in the middle of the night if I was up with a stomachache or some similar affliction. On one particular night, the discomfort was bad enough that I shuffled out of my room into the darkness of the house. Standing at the bottom of the stairs in my nightdress, I whisper-yelled tentatively up towards my parent's bedroom door. My mom sleepily navigated her way down the dark steps toward me and simply stated *go back to sleep, there is nothing I can do*.

Bravery, as I'd learned it, meant not being overcome with emotion in the face of pain: no complaining, no public tears, no neediness. Bravery meant not making my situation anyone else's problem - so even though I had friends all around me at shows, potlucks and groups I felt isolated in what I was going through. I hated how talking about my back made me feel boring, depressing, and weak and instead deferred to silence or fakery. The fact that I appeared healthy on the outside shielded me from questions and camouflaged me against the reality of what was happening inside. Denial for bravery's sake was a mode of survival that allowed me to keep my self-image largely unchanged in the face of injury and I would have kept on that way if not for all of the energy and effort it required, if pain hadn't broken down my ability to concentrate, if it hadn't begun to show on my face and in the way I walked.

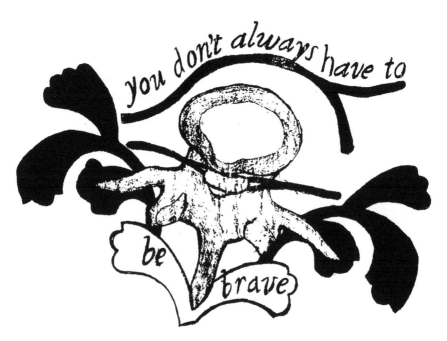

It was maybe the first clear night so far that spring and people were out in dense clusters, pouring into the streets between galleries, clutching dixie cups of red wine from art openings. A group of friends and I had decided to join in on Portland's first

Thursday art walk craziness trekking from Milk Bar to Reading Frenzy and wider off into the newness called The Pearl District, peeking in places along the way. As the night drew on my walking became more labored and concentrated, I was having trouble keeping up with my friends. Months of injury had gotten me used to being at the back of the pack but my muscles were tightening up against each step I took and I was starting to fall behind in earnest. The sidewalks were crowded and navigating the hurried and the tipsy left me feeling even more slow and vulnerable. A loud group of guys were coming towards me and I passed carefully between them, accidentally brushing up against one with my bag. Waiting until he was safely past me the dude I'd made unintentional contact with looked over his shoulder and shouted *Watch where you are going, Hunchback!* and I looked down, flushing with the shame of being exposed. Cruel as it may have been, it wasn't his choice of words that dug into me but rather that my weakness was visible. I was without protection.

It is interesting to me that the word *patient* is both a noun and an adjective. A word that defines a person who is being given medical treatment and simultaneously qualifies them as *able to endure waiting or delay without becoming annoyed or upset.* To be *patient* is *to persevere calmly when faced with difficulties* and to be *able to tolerate being hurt provoked or annoyed without complaint or loss of temper.*

For a year I passed from exam room to exam room seeing countless doctors, acupuncturists, chiropractors, naturopaths, physical therapists, and imaging specialists. Doctors were all saying the same thing: that the choices I had were to continue treating my injury with conservative care and hope for it to heal or to schedule a surgery. Friends and family gave me advice, xeroxed medical articles about the spine and sent them in the mail, offered to drive me to appointments. I took a break from work, which lead to a longer break, which lead to me leaving the job entirely. I felt guilty for needing to spend more and more time in bed, frustrated that no matter what I did things seemed to stay the same or gradually become worse. I was turning 25 in six months time and would no longer be covered by my father's health insurance and I was unable to work for my own. I decided that I had given all that I could to conservative treatment options and resigned myself to back surgery.

For me, deciding on surgery felt more like a failure than a resolution. I felt terrible for being unable to heal on my own. Medically, though I'd searched and researched as much as I had the energy to, I didn't really know what I believed in. I felt pressured to make a decision by the people who cared about me and were weary from seeing me in pain, by the strong feelings they held about different types of medicine, by the success stories they each had to back up their beliefs, by the clock that ticked down my insurance coverage with each passing day, by the self-assurance my doctors and surgeon exuded that theirs was the best course of action. In some ways the validation that surgery offered was enticing. Needing surgery proved that what I had been going through was serious, but I was skeptical that my doctors were hearing my questions and looking at me as an individual. I've come to realize I was correct to question the risks, failures, possible outcomes and possibility for re-injury years after the procedure.

I had to be at the hospital at 6am on the morning of my surgery. I remember changing into a worn flowered gown and sleepily laying in a hospital room with my mother. A nurse came in to start my IV and, with a calm voice and direct look, asked if I was scared. I hadn't really given much thought to fear but tears slipped from my eyes when she questioned me. At that moment, tired and on the verge of getting wheeled into the operating room, I felt like I was finally letting go. Letting go of bravery, letting go of the self-imposed idea that it wasn't ok to fully feel what I'd been feeling for so long, releasing the energy it took to fight what was happening to me, becoming present in the body I had at that moment. I was calm, but sad for myself and a little scared too.

A voice - *The doctor said that you might want this* - accompanied by the feeling of something plastic being placed in my palm, fingers automatically curling to balance what I now held, is the first thing I remember when waking from surgery. My foggy eyes opened, trying to focus on what I'd been given: a clear cup with a blue twist-on lid, my name, birth date, surgeon's name and some numbers printed on a hospital label affixed to its side, a yellow sticker reading *CAUTION: contains formaldehyde* warned me against opening this small strange gift. As I brought the container in for a closer look I discovered two pale pieces of gristly tissue floating within it, the error that had been inside me now in front of my eyes. I couldn't believe the size of it. This great big disruption that I had worked so hard to be bigger than, that had torn through me and turned my life on its head now revealed itself to me in actual size: two diminished bits and an incision the size of a buttonhole.

※※※

After the surgery things got better, but never all the way. Relief from the nerve pain that had been leaving me crooked and crying was such an amazing treat that it took me a while to notice that things were far from perfect. I felt hopeful that total recovery, though slow, would come to me eventually and was thankful for the increased mobility my surgery afforded me.

I threw myself into graduate school applications. Hours in bed had brought me back to books and writing and, since I couldn't work, being a student sounded just about right. I wasn't conscious of this at the time but now I think that going to back to school was a way for me to prove that I had made something of my injury, that pain had led me to a better place in my life and that it had all been worth it. I think I needed to believe that, in this way, pain had been a positive force and that I could begin to distance myself from it by giving it a little triumphant place as part of my story. This romanticized notion was just another attempt at bravery because pain, in lower levels, remained a part of my everyday life.

※※※

There was a certain amount of pain with which I had learned to live without disruption. *Better* became my favorite word, a word that bore the relief of improvement, spoken from the low side of the pain scale diagram. For years, even though the pain persisted, I clung to the idea that I'd been given my solution in surgery. Incomplete though it was, I convinced myself that I was living my recovery and the pain that I felt daily would become less and less until it ceased completely. I chalked my bad days up to poor decision-making and told myself, through the worry those days brought, that each one would be the last.

I didn't identify as a chronic pain patient until seven years into my injury when things became acute for the second time. The signs of re-injury were all too familiar and I felt instantly defeated. Where depression had taken months to sink in last time around, this time I plummeted quickly into hopelessness because I had been down this exact road with injury once before. This time there was no camouflage, the severity of my pain showed: I was pale, I would sweat from trying, and I couldn't manage the basics like tying my shoes or brushing my hair. Everyone's first response was to ask me what I had done - *did I lift something heavy? was I not being careful?* - and because self-neglect had been part of my coping mechanism in the past I beat myself up with blame over the pain I was feeling.

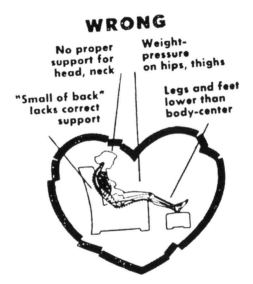

WRONG

No proper support for head, neck

Weight-pressure on hips, thighs

"Small of back" lacks correct support

Legs and feet lower than body-center

The paperwork and self-advocacy required for dealing with my injury, and the ramifications pain had on my work life seemed insurmountable in my depressed and pained state. I'd been turned loose by all of my doctors in the years of relative health after my surgery and had no one who I trusted to see when things became worse. It felt like I was starting over but older, weaker, more worn down from experience. My situation was exactly the same and, at the same time, more complicated entirely.

There were new doctors and familiar tests, fuzzy-making pain medicines, nights on end without sleeping, referrals for a second surgery, a breakthrough with a chiropractor that returned me to work and filled me with hope... then, after that, came the worst days. I remember a sadness that went on for weeks, telling those closest to me between sobs that *I just don't feel like a person,* trying to express how blank and invisible persistent pain can make someone feel. Me, I felt erased because even though I had pared back my commitments consistently over years, I was again unable to do the things I felt defined me. Now pain defined me, and literally immobilized me, and it felt like everything I had done to survive in the past just led me right back to this crisis.

When our neighbors hired a church group to come and tear out the trees that were leading squirrels and other animals onto their roof I got a knock at my front door. Some workers from the group wanted to know if they could come into our back yard to gather the branches they had loosened and catch falling debris from the large trees that backed up to our fence. They wanted to know if there was anything that they should be especially careful of.

I made my way around the house, leading them into our yard. Straight away I became embarrassed by the state of things back there: bushes and vines fighting for sunlight pouring over the rock wall surrounding our garden beds, weeds and grasses up to their work boot's highest eyelet in the space that should have been lawn. Though I dream of wild flowers and growing my own kitchen herbs and vegetables I hadn't been capable of the bending yard work required for seasons. I felt the shame of not wanting to explain how I'd let the plants go untamed, and stood there quietly as they quoted me a price I couldn't afford for work I felt I should be able to do myself. To answer their original question, I gestured toward the only thing I really cared about in our yard, a medium sized dogwood tree planted square in the center that blooms a delicate pink every spring. They nodded towards the tree promising to be aware of it, handed me their cards in case I changed my mind about needing their services, and went back around the house to get to work.

When I no longer heard voices or chainsaws I peered out the window at our yard, now strangely out of context without its backdrop, and saw my favorite tree accidentally broken down in the center.

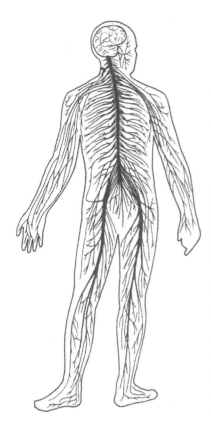

In my experience, pain brings with it a flow of questions and difficulties that seem bottomless. We look to health practitioners for answers. We look inward for causes, for strength, and hope. Along with physical discomfort, pain brings fear, doubt, urgency, loss and anger and, if it persists, pain gives these feelings time to root in and grow wild.

In the past I've met these challenges with a defense of bravery. I've voluntarily suffered the definition of what it means to be a patient. I have denied the long-term nature of my injury, searching for ways to get over it without ever looking at it directly.

Now I think it is brave to meet my injury squarely as fact, to work on accepting pain as part of my identity, to give myself space to be honest about what I've been through and mourn losses, to reach out to people and create community around pain, to make a point to write and talk about it even when it makes me feel self-conscious, boring or weak, to search out health practices I believe in and practitioners that listen, to work on my tendency toward catastrophic thinking, to try and find a place of rest and honor for my worst days ever, to ask for help and accept it, to devote myself to swimming and other things that feel good and give me power, to take time out to be thankful and amazed by the healing process and all of the other things my body knows how to do, to dream dreams from the body I have now and not save my hopes and desires until I am well, to realize that I may never be well but keep fighting for the care and visibility I deserve.

It is July of 2008, the beginning of my ninth year as a person in pain. I am lying in bed as I write this, propped up by pillows in all the learned places. This spring brought with it the fragile beauty of dogwood blooms. Despite the splitting of a branch that held a third of its growth our tree is producing new leaves, proof of what it is capable of - the ability to survive its losses.

a conversation about chronic pain

Cassandra (b. 1981) and Shelby (b. 1992) had the fortunate experience of meeting in 2002 when Shelby's dad was dating Cassandra. For the next four years, they spent every summer and several other holidays together. Instead of disliking each other, they became the best of friends. After Cassandra and Shelby's dad broke up, they remained friends.

Cassandra: We met when you were 10, almost 11. At what point did you realize I had a condition(s) that caused chronic pain?

Shelby: I thought it was just part of you. It didn't occur to me it was chronic pain; it just seemed an innate aspect of your being. When my dad first sort of said anything, two years into knowing you, was the first time I realized you were more than just sickly.

C: Would you name some examples of when you think my having chronic pain limited the activities of our relationship?

S: We never had full day excursions and I remember you would get sick if we tried to go anywhere far on the bus or in the car.

C: Did your dad ever discuss or explain my condition(s) or chronic pain in general to you?

S: When we first got to Australia, he had a talk with me. We all had jet lag, but you were sleeping during the day too. He told me I couldn't really bother you during the day, that I had to be quiet and not cause you too much trouble.

I remember walking around a lot with you guys, not, like, far or anything. We did a lot, I thought, at the time.

He was pretty insensitive, or he would make a lot of remarks that I wouldn't relate to how you always seemed to be feeling under the weather. He just indicated that he thought there was always something wrong with you. I feel like he resented it.

C: Did you ever worry or wonder if it was something you would "catch" or develop from being around me?

S: I remember once [when I was 11] you carried me over a puddle on the way to a department store. I remember you explaining to me some of the illnesses you had in high school. I didn't feel like you were contagious or anything, I just remember thinking, "*oh, so that explains some of it.*" Feeling like a revelation, almost. But like I said, I never really felt like it made a big difference, because at the time I didn't notice, like at the time I just thought it was part of you, just who you were.

C: Did you ever think I was faking it for whatever reason? (Be honest; I've heard it from everyone and can take it!) If so, for what reason?

S: I don't think you were ever faking it, but I do remember towards the end of the relationship [between you and my father] I was having a lot of mixed emotions. Like, when you two would argue, I would flip back and forth between his side and your side, and think "*Why is he being so harsh on her?*" and "*Why are you being so hypercritical of him?*" It occurred to me a few times that you exaggerated [your health] a lot. And I kinda sided with him for a few occasions when he was like, "*You just don't want to do anything,*" not making it up but exaggerating your condition. But that was during the worst part of it. I remember being really emotionally confused and stressed.

C: How did you perceive how your dad acted/acknowledged the situation/me regarding my health, specifically the pain?

S: He has this tendency where he thinks he's comforting but instead if feels like he's humoring you. Every now and then, if you were laying down he would just go over and pat you on the head and say, "*Awww,*" like, it didn't feel like he took it very seriously and I got the sense that he resented it all.

C: It was really hard for me because he and I both have sciatica. When he would have a sciatic flare, he would be down on the ground, flat and moaning and be an absolute bear - you've seen him do this. When I would have a sciatic flare, he would just be like, "*come on, keep going, let's go*," for me, it had to be, pat me on the head, just another one of my problems, but for him it had to be the end of the world.

S: He's not every empathetic to others. He's more paranoid about keeping me healthy so that my mother doesn't get mad at him than he is for the sake of keeping me healthy, because he's sent me home sick so many times.

C: What's your understanding of my condition—specifically what causes the chronic pain - and how it limits me, now that you're so very much older? ;)

S: I guess the real difference is that now I don't see it as being part of you, I see it has being a real medical condition. I know a lot of it can be triggered by anxiety - I talked to my doctors about it and they told me about how it can be somatoform, or psychologically. Not that I didn't take it seriously before, but now I have a different perception of it. And I realize it's not a part of who you are, even though you've been coping with it for so long, from what I understand, the majority of your life.

C: I know I've explained all of it over the years to you, but I guess you've remembered bits and pieces. So, your understanding of it is that it's more of a somatic pain than - I mean, I actually have a spine deformity - but you apparently don't remember me telling you about that part?

S: I remember about the bone spurs on your butt.

C: Yeah, that's what causes the most pain. 'Cause it pinches off a nerve. But the rest of it, as you said, can be linked to, I mean, any pain can be linked to an emotional or environmental setting or whatnot.

You recently told both your father and me that you have a cyst in one of your ovaries. That leads to my next couple of questions.

I started having gynecological problems with severe pain as a teenager, too. How has it affected your experience as a teenager?

S: I found that when I told some of my friends that I had a cyst and that it was causing lots of pain - before I realized what it was, I was getting really snappish and extremely irritable and I thought I was PMSing but I wasn't. And my period would never come and I would have lots of anxiety, which

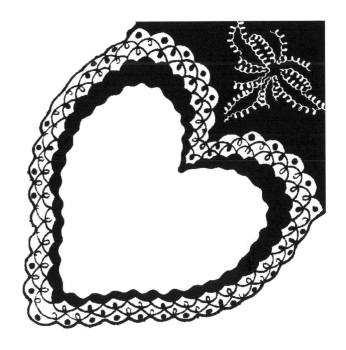

would irritate me further. So when I told them what I had, it's not that they didn't take it seriously, but... they turned it into a running joke, like, "*Oh, your cyst is acting up again.*"

A lot of the time when I'm hanging out with people whom I feel really comfortable with, I ask them to press down on my lower back or on my lower tummy in the front, like if I'm watching tv or movies. It doesn't really affect my swimming. It makes me paranoid, though, because of the spotting, I think it's my period but it's not, so I go to the bathroom a lot, thinking I'm bleeding everywhere, which can be annoying because my teachers can be like, "*Why are you going to the bathroom all the time?*"

When it comes to relationships, [sexually] I've been giving more than receiving; just because of how sensitive I am, which seems really unfair. They want to reciprocate but it's hard for me to let them... but it doesn't always bother me.

C: How did your father react when you told him about the cyst, and why do you think he acted in that manner?

S: When I told him he was surprised, and then he got really angry because I hadn't told him. The way he found out was because I had to go to the gynecologist for an intra-vaginal sonogram the next day. Then he was like, "*Well, when did THIS happen, because you never told me, your mother never said anything...*"

C: Because your seventeen-year-old vagina is his property and his business? [both laughing]

S: Yeah, and he immediately after being angry he got very awkward about it. "*Don't you worry, everything will be fine, get that taken care of now [pet name].*" Like, he never even mentioned, "*How does that make you feel, is it uncomfortable?*" - like before, how I mentioned, it's like how he doesn't take care of me to prevent sickness for the sake of keeping me healthy and happy, it's like [he's doing it to keep from being in trouble.] Like he doesn't have a reaction a father should have. I'm of the opinion that, "*You're my father, swallow your fear! I don't need a fake response.*" I'd be much happier, I think, without anything. I'd be happier with a sincere response than with nothing.

C: One of the things I've dealt with is having polycystic ovarian syndrome - now just because you have one cyst, it doesn't mean you have PCOS, so don't freak out. But if your doctor did diagnose you with PCOS, how do you anticipate that impacting upon your life?

S: Um. Negatively, I think.

C: Well, it doesn't have to have a huge negative impact.

S: Well, I can't foresee, really, because I'm not sure how my body would react if I had to take yucky medications all the time. But just from the pain perspective, and I guess psychologically, it would be difficult, because I'm always staying up late, I'm always working on something. I anticipate the next four years [of college] to be a huge strain and very stressful. When I sleep, it's easier, but if I don't sleep, it hurts a lot more.

C: As two gorgeous young ladies with chronic pain, how do you envision a future for us, with us, while we still have pain?

S: I love to knit and crochet, so I want to maybe make beautiful heating pad and hot water bottle covers - they're all so ugly!

C: Don't forget, you still have to design a floating, all-encompassing sphere to protect my butt with. It'll be the bustle of the twenty-first century.

S: Right!

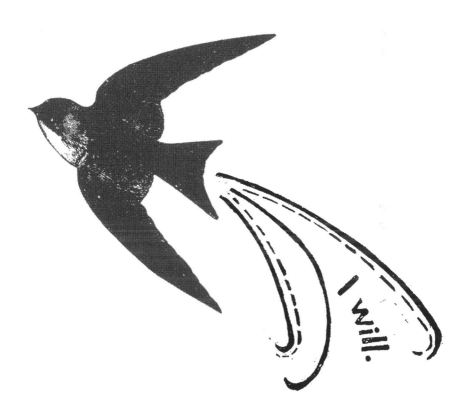

Marissa Raguet

chronic illness,
painful childhood

When I was 7 years old I started feeling the pain. Being that
it was the early 90s, I naturally envisioned small PAC-MANs
slowly gnawing their way through my intestine. They were a
dull roar brought out almost every time I ate and often even if
I didn't. My father had similar pain, the result of Crohn's, an
inflammatory bowel disease. I still remember my mother telling
me the day before I was to see the doctor for tests that I couldn't
have Crohn's, that everything was fine. I wasn't even curious to
know, I just wanted the pain to stop. The pain itself is like a black
hole: it's an orange sunset early Fall evening and we're eating
dinner together as we always do: my dad, mom, older sister,
older brother, and I. Conversation turns from work, to school,
to neighbors, to future events as we savor a green salad with
tomato and ranch dressing, baked potato with cheese, canned
heavy syrup peaches, and grilled steak with BBQ sauce. I take
much less food, eat more slowly, and savor it more. I chatter
almost non-stop about what I'm learning in science class and
a book I'm loving. I've made it through the salad and peaches,
and I start to feel the familiar dull roar - like a large and jagged
coal, soft and hot, starting somewhere near the beginning of my
large intestine and being forced by peristalsis slowly through
to the end. It sucks my energy inward as my body puts all of its
resources towards attending to that area. It steals my voice: I
become distracted and silent. It steals my hunger: I stop eating
and start pretending to eat. My body re-centers itself around
the place of pain - I hunch over and wrap my arms warmly and
gently around my waist. I leave the food, the chatter, and the
sunset, and lie on my bed on my side with my knees pulled to my
chest, my door closed to outside distraction which would require
energy I don't have. The black hole of pain requires it all.

Five years of this pain and Crohn's and my body looks the part.
It's 1995 and I'm standing in front of my parents' full-length
bathroom mirror staring at a body that doesn't resemble me.

This malnutritioned body - so short, so thin, so stunted - isn't me. My body looks 9 years old. But I've lived for 12 years. And my wise mind - my actual self - I feel, is somewhere in her 80s. At the time, I feel I know what someone in his/her 80s knows - the important things in life, and the closeness of death. My anguish over the reminder of having this body is too much. I lie in bed and pray - for inches; even just three more would make me somewhat more normal and thus make me happy. I pleaded to have a normal body like those my friends had. As I got older I matured in my understanding of the truth about Crohn's. PAC-MEN weren't real, but DNA mutations passed down by my parents' genes were. My own body was my enemy - literally programmed from the start for failure. In high school Biology class I learned how small DNA was; I daydreamed taking tweezers and rearranging every Crohn's mutation in every cell in my body. It seemed strange to me that I could know what was wrong, but be unable to communicate this to my body so that it could make the appropriate adjustments. What's the point of having a body if we can't even talk, if we can't be reliable friends? For all of these reasons, my body wasn't me, and I had little care for it.

As bad as a physical pain and mental anguish of the illness itself were, negative interactions more so defined my childhood. These memories are like magician's knives; no matter how many times I pull them out of my heart, the next time I look they're always back again, and bloody: an older kid on the school bus who told me and those sitting around us that people like me shouldn't be allowed to attend school. A family friend who asked how old I was and then was so shocked by my answer that she demanded I tell her the truth. An older kid who confronted me in the school hallway and told me he was going to pick me up and throw me like a football. A friendly classmate who when told he should date me responded with, "No way, she reminds me of my little sister." A stranger touring campus with his family who yelled at me from across the street, "Hey, how old are you!?" A girl at another school who came up to me during lunch to ask my age and then ran back and told those at her table, who then all turned towards me and stared and whispered quietly. It was a scene in my life repeated often: "You're a freak!" proceeded by accusatory staring and silence.

Crohn's caused a physical pain
that often silenced my words
as the pain drew my focus and
energy inward. And it caused
a mental anguish because it
made my body into something I
couldn't relate to or love. But it
was these negative interactions
with the people mentioned above
that caused an upending that
often silenced my soul. I didn't
need for everyone to know that
I had Crohn's and offer their
utmost support; I just needed
people to not be careless with
their questions or directly cruel.
To heal, in my mind I create
a different world and as my
younger self wander those
school hallways, city streets,
and family reunions. In school,
a teenage boy runs up to me,
gives me a light hug, and asks
how I'm feeling today. At a
family reunion, a relative I don't
recognize asks me what grade
I'm in and after my response
excitedly asks about my favorite
subject. On the city streets, many
of us freaks are out strolling
tonight. Some of the normal
people smile and say good
evening as they do to everyone
they pass, but the rest just
remain engrossed in their own
lives and leave us to ourselves.

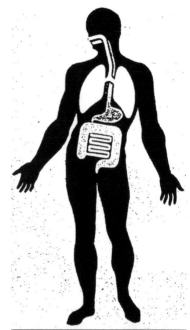

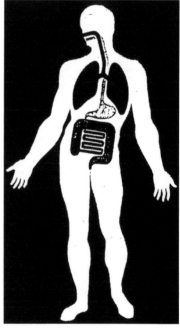

Jonah Aline Daniel

a love letter to **my** *arms*

this is numb
this is avoiding
ignoring
forgetting
not listening
this is numb

today while i was walking home after a hard arm day,
i appreciated out loud how well my legs worked

this must be a love letter to my arms i said
this will be a love letter to my hands

a lorazepam taken earlier assuages the panic, the betrayal that
lives there these days
and a love letter to my arms emerges. a love letter to my hands

on tuesday in a moment when six things needed to happen
urgently, aurora calls out "with your other two hands, will you
do such and such..." i don't have ANY hands i say out loud to
myself. we decide i must figure out why i don't have hands.
where they've gone and for what reason. what the demands of
the strike are and under what conditions the labor negotiations
must take place.

this is tingling
these swollen tissues
aching joints
this is stagnation
this is inflammation
this is anxiety, panic, stuckness
this is tingling

a love letter to my hands. how unappreciated they've been
how thanklessly they've labored
how hard they've worked

swimming in lake michigan all day until the sun sets - summer
after summer
and learning to swim in the chlorine filled tiled and echoey pool
as a tiny one on saturday mornings at the high school
blueberry picking and cherry picking and peach picking with
mom and dad year after year
all the orgasms they've give me in the last 11 years -
thousands.
volleyball and track training setting and hitting, push-ups and
weightlifting
book making smoothing and punching and cutting sewing
and cooking - chopping and stirring and kneading folding, with
appropriate and inappropriate tools lifting cast irons and big
heavy pots

sleeping on my side on floors and hard surfaces, waking to numb
limbs, climbing ladders

massages for friends before training - bent back and twisted
neck, all thumbs and fingers
and a hundred hours of massage training learning technicals
and nothing about the sacred of this work. my body is a machine
to make money for myself or someone else, i learn.

this is dead empty bored and far away

middle school, high school, college - stooped back slouched in the
chair.
hundreds of hours of copying history book lies in outlines on
lined paper
writing filled with procrastination, perfectionism, pressure and
regurgitation
7 years of laptop claws typing
of course the urgent texting

this is dead empty bored and far away
where have i gone and what do i need to live in my body?

a year of caretaking, of dishwashing, hand washing clothes,
lifting buckets and watering cans, screwing in screws,
hammering nails, sweeping and cutting vegetables, depending

on my hands for making money. using my arms and hands to
facilitate the health of someone else's body.

i put my hands on my dad's aching cancer filled head this visit.
my body shaking with sobs he couldn't see. i even ordered a book
called medicine hands: massage therapy for people with cancer...

i used to pull at the hanging skin on my grandma's arms
and hands
i liked it. it was so strange to me and so grotesque and
fascinating and lovely to see all of those veins and bones and that
old skin hanging from her body
i used my hands to call the ambulance when she fell in
february
in that er held her hand and her head as they poked her and
prodded her and struggled to find a vein in her dehydrated 75
pound body

in that icu i helped move her arm so her broken wrist and
balloon hand could be elevated. i got to hold her hand with my
hand before she died.

this is dissociation
this is stiff stuck claw hands
this is clumsy knocking everything over

cash registers
photography chemicals
caress
hands submerged in huge bowls of flax
stimulating onion tops in a green house
grateful for all the things i can feel
how will i find my use without these hands

and injuries as well
a fall facilitated by a drunken friend takes part of a finger when i
catch a bicycle pedal on the way to the ground
furious chopping takes the top of a thumb and a dull knife sweet
potato accident slices all the way down that same thumb
and the burns—reaching for pots and into ovens and grills with
bare hands, i joke i never obtained that learning curve about hot

this is invisible
pain that no one can see
hands that cramp and curl at the sight of someone who
might notice
remember help sympathize care

this is invisible
illness no one can see
this is eyes swimming in a crazy raging head
intentional scratching at wrists now too faint to make out by
anyone but me.
more desperation than death wish

this is
maam
she her miss lady girl
sister daughter girlfriend

and man dude brother mister sir
see me my arms cry out

this is invisible
helplessness despair terror panic hopelessness
pain that no one can see
see me my arms cry out

this is numb
this is avoiding
ignoring
forgetting
not listening
this is numb

sustained yoga postures, holding, watching those creases in my
wrists, twisting and sweating - what relief and release and peace
it's brought me

and the rage and grief that's left my body through punching bags

and then there are those really stressful times - not mistakes
exactly but beyond the call of duty for sure. like riding 1100

miles on someone else's pace and with all my weight resting on
those terrible handlebars
and those time i've tried to fist myself. i'm really sorry about that
wrists.

i've been so angry at you but i feel it softening. ive felt so
betrayed but i understand more now about why you are leaving
me. i've felt such intense panic - how could i ever survive without
you in this world - without you arms and hands. how cruel i am
even now - you have to work and hurt for your own love letter as
i write this. i will do whatever you ask. i love you.

this is numb
this is avoiding
ignoring
forgetting
not listening
this is numb
it's worth noticing when you can't feel and ask why

this is stranded
this is alone
this is forced to stay in one place
if i won't choose it my body will insist upon it

this is tingling
these swollen tissues
aching joints
this is stagnation
this is inflammation
this is anxiety, panic, stuckness
this is a reminder of life in tiny prickly bursts

on intersecting pain

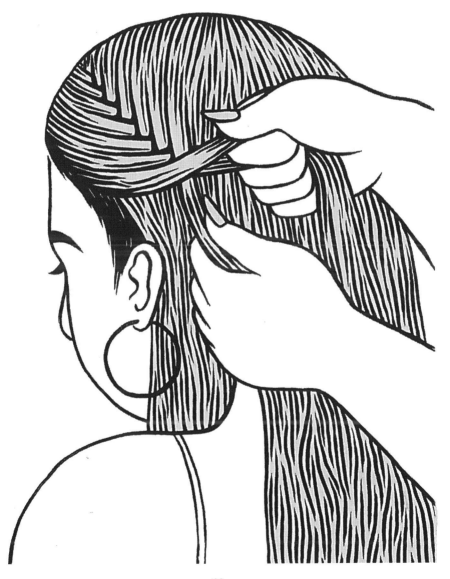

before trigger warnings

The hip pain came on suddenly in 2009. Maybe it was always there and I was too busy working full time, going to school full time, and nursing mine and others' addictions to notice it. Or maybe the adrenaline of my teens, early, and mid-twenties brought on by survival and assimilation staved it off. 2009 was the year that my mom after thirty-five years, got a restraining order on my dad and left him. I slid into being her main support person, full of resolve and might. I talked to her on the phone more than I ever had, listening to her recount her traumatic experiences, many of them decades old, and tried to get them to flow through me, but their sediment attached to my walls. A few months went by, she focused on her job and healing her heart. And then she went back. My hips gave way. I was in so much pain I couldn't sleep on my side. Six years later, the pain flows steadily like an IV drip.

Some things are facts. My dad grew up as a Navy brat and lived in places as far away from each other as Alaska and Guam. At the end of his senior year, his family moved from California to Rhode Island and his new school had different graduation requirements. The administrators told him he had to attend an extra year to get his diploma. He said, "Fuck it," and volunteered for Vietnam so he could pick his duty and avoid being disowned by his military family. His dad and brother had already toured Vietnam twice together putting electrical lines and poles up and now it was his turn. My dad became a heavy equipment operator, driving big trucks and building houses out of sandbags. That's where he got sprayed with Agent Orange.

As the war went on, like his peers, Dad and his friends believed in it less and less and, to cope, used more and more drugs. Pot, morphine, binoctal, heroin. They say one in five U.S. soldiers in Vietnam used heroin. The night before his return to his hometown San Diego, after serving his year in the war, he and his buddies got set up on their way back to the base. Their car was searched and the planted drugs were found in the glove box. Instead of heading back home, he was flown from Vietnam to

Seattle, tried and sentenced to six months in a military prison scrubbing asbestos out of the hulls of ships. He was nineteen and no longer eligible for Veteran's benefits.

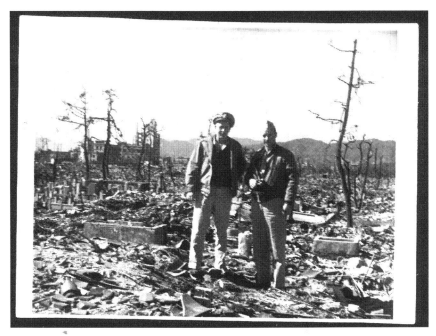

THE AUTHOR'S GREAT-GRANDFATHER (LEFT) AND FELLOW SOLDIER IN HIROSHIMA AFTER THE U.S. BOMBING

Is it Dad's time in war why I avoid being out in the woods and why I spend most days worrying if someone will shoot me in the back? Is it Dad's exposure to six months of asbestos or his exposure to Agent Orange the reason I am allergic to fresh paint, nail polish, hair spray, mold, dust, grass, and gluten? Is it Dad's exposure to six months of asbestos or his exposure to Agent Orange the reason I have chronic muscular, joint, and myofascial pain all over my body? Is it Dad's lifetime of drug use that caused my own drug and alcohol addiction? Me and all of my siblings. What caused the birth defects? The inability to conceive? The nightmares? The poverty?

Beat poet David Meltzer says, "write about the pain without showing the wound." For awhile there in kindergarten and first grade, soon after I got my first bike, anytime I fell off it and got a scrape, Mom and Dad would hold me down with glee and douse me with what they called, "Monkey's Blood". Their grip was the opposite of how I felt right before falling, my feet hovering above the pedals, eyes closed, hair whipping behind me, my hands flirting with letting go of the handlebars. While the Monkey's Blood sting was unbearable, I was most upset by the possibility that actual monkey's blood was on me. With each cut or scrape they kept holding me down, dousing me, refusing to assure me this liquid wasn't actually blood from an actual monkey. Mercurochrome. That's its real name. An old fashioned over-the-counter remedy that's since been banned by the FDA due to its mercury content.

These are also the facts. I can't remember the last time my dad went to a doctor; fifteen years, maybe twenty. He prides himself on it. Not on being not sick or not in pain, but on being sick or in pain and not asking for help. He's outlived his father by four years already, so something is working.

There's a picture of Dad in Vietnam kneeling with a group of kids, he's eighteen and they're eight or nine. All of them eat rice from bowls and look up into the camera. Starting twelve years later, he never knelt with me like that. Instead, he let his childhood terrorize me. He tried to freeze me in his trauma triangle, and for a long time, succeeded. Us, bouncing from one town to the next and then back again, me attending twenty-five schools before graduating high school. Maybe he couldn't bend his knees. I'm glad at least those Vietnamese kids got to have him there and I can see now that at one time he could be with them, then.

My dad can hardly walk now. After a visit last summer, I searched for free chiropractic services. Thirty minutes from his house, there is a church that on Wednesdays from 7-9p.m. hosts a free drop-in chiropractic clinic. I told my mom to tell my dad. He didn't go.

I wouldn't put it past my dad to be responsible for my hip pain. At least in part. The line of years of his men I kept out of me with the power of my hips circles around an unknown planet. "Have you ever considered that there may be a connection between your hip pain and sexual trauma?" a beloved acupuncturist once asked me as she tried to get some movement between my femur and my pelvis. What good is it, putting language to something the body already knows?

Really the only difference between me and my dad is I got access to healing he didn't get access to. He's tried lots of outdated home remedies. All the drugs including the hard ones. Shot gun when not at the pawnshop, in the mouth. Before trigger warnings. Things I'll never know about. How many times can you threaten suicide before it's decided you're a coward? How many times can you pawn a thing before it loses its value?

The consequence of our difference is my audience is bigger than his, bigger than a dark-filled room in the rainforest, sleep broken by Agent Orange sweats, the only ticket holders a helpless daughter and a desperate wife. I traded in the isolation I inherited. I haven't quite figured out how to reach for him, but I can finally reach for almost all of myself. I have tasted life without suffering and it tastes glorious.

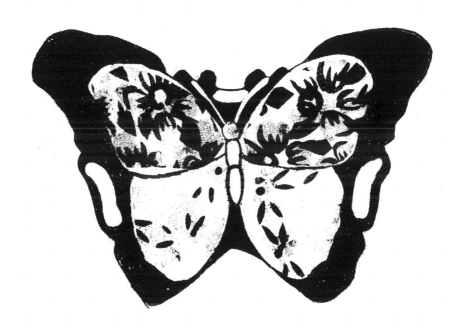

mama in pain

If not for the danger of electrocution, I would be writing this from my bathtub. That little ceramic container of warmth has become a refuge for me that I retreat to one to two times daily. Since my daughter, Paloma, was born 11 months ago it's been one of the few places I can be totally alone. It's a safe, quiet place I can sink into myself and reflect. It's also one of my most effective painkillers since being pregnant and then breastfeeding and caring for a child have significantly reduced my options in that category. I like the encompassing pressure of the water against my skin. Its simultaneous softness and weight calm the buzzing of my over-stimulated nerves and relax the defensive grip of my muscles. At the end of each day, when my pain and exhaustion tend to peak, I can't wait to get in the bath.

In fact, Paloma was born in warm water. I had planned a water birth in our home, and when the time came I was eager for the midwives to give me the go ahead to jump in the tub. By then my contractions were going strong and there was a powerful ache in my lower back and pelvis as my baby's little body continued to move down. The water supported me and it also provided a sweet transition for Paloma as she left the womb and entered the world.

In every way, the pain of labor was the opposite of my chronic pain experience. Amazing hormones of joy obviously had an influence. But to begin with, the very foundation of the pain was opposite. While my chronic pain was evidence of trauma and malfunction, the pain of labor was caused by the incredible transformation of my body as it produced life. There was and would be no injury. While with my chronic pain I normally felt fear and disconnection from my physical self, during labor I felt a complete trust of and love for my body and its innate abilities. I was grounded inside myself, present, feeling the power of the pain of my contractions as they did their work.
After Paloma was born I was sure I would be able to hold onto those feelings of fearlessness and connection to my body.

Unfortunately, it wasn't so easy. During my pregnancy I had for the most part experienced a lessening of my pain. Post baby, my pain has returned, though somewhat altered. I don't actually feel all the time how I felt during labor, but my memory of it is an awesome reference that I feel lucky to access when I'm really struggling with my pain.

I knew before getting pregnant that parenting with chronic pain would pose challenges. So far I have only had time to experience what challenges exist for the mother of a very young person. Struggling with those challenges, I began to wonder how my mother had coped with having major depression while she raised my sister and myself, and decided to ask her about it.

"I found being around you guys to be helpful when I was feeling depressed," my mom told me on the phone. "In the beginning I didn't suffer from post partum depression, I suffered from post partum ecstasy." We both laughed. I asked her how she found ways to not take out her depression on us when we were older.

"When you were old enough I explained my depression to you in age-appropriate terms," she said. "Mostly I didn't struggle with depression around you guys. I did get into psychotherapy and also that was around when Prozac first came out." My mom did tell me about a time when my sister lived with her and I did not, when she became very depressed after she split with her partner of 5 years. They went on a road trip together to lift her spirits but it didn't work.

"On the ride home I just felt so dead and flat, and I said to your sister, 'I just feel like I'm looking out at a desert and there is no oasis in sight' and your sister said to me 'I'll be your oasis mom' and it was so touching, but I knew she shouldn't have to be my oasis. But that's how it was, I was depressed." My mom cried a little telling me this story. It made me think of times when I've been short tempered with my baby because of my pain, and the guilt I feel after. And it reminded me that we have to know we are doing the best we can and our children will still thrive.

I certainly haven't experienced the post partum ecstasy my mother did, although there have been many moments of joy in this first year of life. One of the biggest challenges I have faced is the lack of sleep and how it affects my body. When I don't sleep well, it seems my body never relaxes enough to get a break and heal. I have been blessed with a child who wakes frequently, even more than most babies I know. That means the next day is worse than the day before. And unfortunately, carrying a heavy object all day long (something I never did before I had a baby) has increased my old pain and created some new spots of trouble in my back and neck. That has a lot to do with nursing as well. More pain means less energy and patience for my daughter and my partner, which I feel is the biggest issue I struggle with as a parent with chronic pain. I just have a shorter fuse. I imagined I would be the most patient parent in the world, and I'm not.

One day when Paloma was around 3 months old, I found myself literally yelling at her because she wouldn't nap. My back was hurting very badly and I was exhausted from waking with her 5 or 6 times a night. Afterward, of course, I felt terrible. It was a wake up call to take more breaks and get more help.

It's not just the deficiency in maternal patience that I have been surprised by. I'm sure nobody's expectations for parenting completely match up with the real deal, but it does seem that parents with chronic illness specifically struggle more with having to give up on a lot of the parenting techniques they wanted to use. At least, that's the impression I got surfing the parenting forum on mothering.com, where there were a few threads for parents with chronic pain and chronic illness. Most of us on this discussion board are believers in attachment style parenting, yet there were so many posts from mamas who had to stop breastfeeding or co-sleeping early because of the pain they experienced, or who couldn't wear their babies in slings for the same reason. Other changes might include less financial stability than anticipated due to doctor's bills or inability to work, less energy and patience for parenting, and decreased mobility which limits things like trips to the park.

There is grief when one has to let go of these desirable gifts one wants to give one's child. I sometimes feel resentful that I spent so many years as a nanny wearing other people's babies and

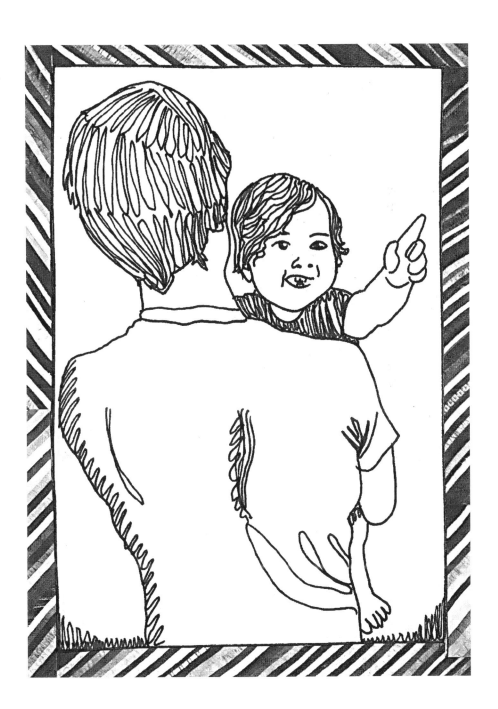

now I can't wear my own for more than 10 minutes. I have also stopped co-sleeping at a much earlier age than I anticipated, because getting my body comfortable enough to sleep is enough of a challenge without adding a squirmy baby into the mix. In addition to grief I feel guilt about denying my child these good things, and find myself at times feeling shame in the presence of other mamas who are parenting a different way.

Like so many other aspects of life with chronic pain, as a parent I've had to redefine what I think of as a successful and fulfilling life. It takes a lot of work to let go of my idealized image of family life. But the more I'm able to do that, the more present I am for my baby, and the more creative I am at replacing the things I wanted with new concepts of parent-child interaction. We can use the stroller instead of the sling and still enjoy our walk. We can play in the pool instead of the park; especially since we both love the water.

More than anything, I don't want these unhelpful feelings to color my daughter's childhood in an unhealthy way. I want to care for myself and work with my feelings so that Paloma doesn't have to carry them for me. I've had to expand and amplify the skill set I've developed as a person with chronic pain. Taking time away from her and talking to people about the hard times helps me with my short temper. Getting friends and family to babysit even for an hour or two gives my body a break from the grunt work of hauling around a child. Making space to be with my body in a positive way, either in the bath or in a dance class, helps me pass on the concepts that our bodies are our wonderful allies, not our adversaries. On a day when I am struggling with a flare up, I sometimes just stop and remember, image by image, those amazing few days when Paloma was born. And I believe that if my body and I can bring forth life, we can find a way to be happy and healthy in this world.

Meredith Butner

skeleton

The structure on the corner
asserts its new shape
with an urgency unusual
to this neighborhood.
Flaunting its work crew
to the nearby Victorian,
left stripped and half-painted
five years, this house,
which sat less than two
mid-ruin, wins every envy
as the language of its
second story arrives.

Now, a week into revision,
fresh two-by-fours outline
a bare suggestion
of floor, roof and room.
These new frames move
the house upward, add height
to those the fire left sturdy,
partition and divide a view
of the sky, imply which space
will be contained, held interior.

House, we all desire to be built
back from our losses so.
Skeleton become scaffold, and soon.

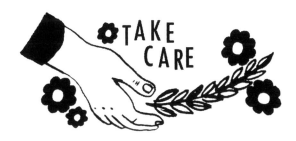

Sunny Drake

capitalism hurts
as if i wasnt hurting enough already

My body and I: one of those old married couples. We are best
friends yet we bicker and struggle with each other every day.
We spend all our time together yet sometimes we discover how
little we really know about the other. Our relationship used to
be built on an understanding that I would call the shots and my
body would keep it up, albeit with occasional grumbles. That
is, until eight months ago when I had a repetitive strain injury
in both my wrists which progressed from acute tendonitis to
chronic pain. Now our dynamic is reversed - my body calls pretty
much all the shots these days. We've been to various "couples
counselors" so to speak, but no one can tell me exactly what is
going on with my body. Anything requiring even a slight grip
or repetitive motions with my hands is difficult. Cooking, riding
a bike, writing, computer work, sex, opening jars, lifting my
bag, going to the toilet and stroking a friend's hair are daily
challenges. With these radical changes in what I can and can't
do, I've found a myriad of ways that I devalue myself and that
others devalue me. Thanks capitalism for that extra hurt, as if I
wasn't hurting enough already.

Before exploring the ways that capitalism has insidiously seeped
into how I view myself and others, it's important to acknowledge
some of my identities that shape my experiences. I am a mixed
class femme queer trans man. I am white, with English and
Irish ancestors, and I was born and grown in Australia. I am a
writer, performer, producer, activist, project manager, friend,
lover, family member, caretaker, and random dancer at traffic
lights and subways. I do not claim to understand what it would
be like to have a longer term or wider reaching disability, or how
the impacts of ableism would magnify if I weren't white. This
injury has given me a small window of insight into the world of
ableism, how it plays out in my own life, as well as in activist
and queer subcultures. This article is based on listening to the
insightful and important experiences of people with disabilities,
the pondering I've done in the quiet moments of despair about

my wrists, and my participation in the Ann Braden anti-racism training for white activists in San Francisco.

How does capitalism hurt? I am realizing just how deep the capitalist mentality is interwoven into how I think, how I value people, and what I base my identity on. The change in my body's functionality has triggered a major shift in my self-identity and I have been struggling with feeling worthless. Every day I find myself thinking: "I'm not doing anything", "I'm not contributing to my community", and justifying my "un-productive" existence by the fact that I have an injury that prevents me from doing "valuable" things. The only way I have been able to feel okay about myself is by framing this period of my life as "healing time," and reassuring myself that at some point I'll be able to do "valuable" work again. This has prompted me to start questioning what I consider "valuable" and what I consider "work".

It is so embedded in my thinking to define only project or organizational activity as "work". Harsha Walia asserts, "Capitalism not only creates the conditions for the expropriation of labour, but also limits what can even be characterized as labour" . Capitalism considers work as activity done outside the domestic or relationship spheres which results in tangible products and outcomes. Walia points out that "work" is also tied to what you extract from the land. When I consider different ideas about work that center emotional labour and relationships, with this injury I am still doing valuable work and contributing to my community. I am a key emotional support person for several people. I listen to people and workshop their relationships challenges. I link people with each other. I share insights from different contexts like relating Australian and U.S. struggles. I am excellent at drawing out the unique and remarkable aspects of the people I meet, and I support others to achieve their goals. I have long chats with friends and random strangers about their lives, hopes, and dreams. I tell stories and create theatre that challenges dominant ideas. I give feedback and encouragement on friend's creative projects. I participate in a collective household. I appreciate calendula flowers almost every day.

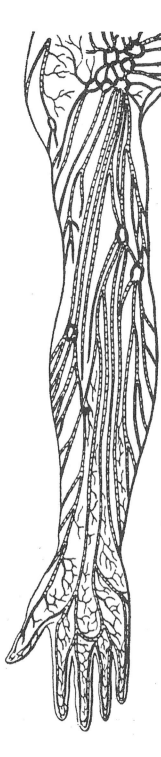

It is no coincidence that most of these undervalued roles are considered feminine or female roles: welcome to the white supremacist colonial capitalist patriarchy. Women and femmes are expected to do this work freely and this labour is neither credited as work nor valued. Hence, people who do this emotional work are also devalued. In a time when we are in serious plight on planet earth, it's not only necessary to start valuing emotional and care work, but in fact centering it. Harsha Walia highlights that care work is necessary to continue life on earth.

So, I don't want to hold out for the day my wrists get better to start feeling good about myself again. By refusing to acknowledge the worth of my own life right now, I am participating in devaluing the worth and lives of so many other people who do not fit able-bodied capitalist norms. I am contributing to driving the planet further into the abyss we are facing.

In addition to what capitalism encourages us to value and devalue, I've also been thinking about how capitalism encourages us to work. Overhauling white supremacist, sexist, capitalist and able-ist systems involves digging deep and changing how we do things. For example, capitalism is obsessed with accelerating profit curves, quick fixes and short-term vision. As activists, when are we uncritically propelling these ways of working? For instance, when are we failing to create deep change by focusing on superficial changes that simply make us look good or get our not-for-profit organizations more funding? Given the urgency of social and environmental issues, it's understandable that many of us have short-term crisis mentalities, rather than working towards strategic bigger visions. But who gets left behind when the focus is on more-faster-have-to-get-it-done-today-or-else? Does a preoccupation with accelerated outcomes lend itself to genuine reflection or simply doing what it takes to make outcomes look good? Some examples of how I see these capitalist mentalities embedded within activist work include:

- Encouraging a culture of work-a-holism that many people with disabilities are unable to participate in.
- "But it was the only meeting space we could find": focus on the easiest logistics such as holding meetings in spaces or at times inaccessible to many people.
- "This campaign is about stopping mining, not gender equality or Indigenous sovereignty": breaking down complex social change issues into single issues. The outcome is ironically a failure to understand the root causes of even those "single" issues, such as how colonization and patriarchy are interwoven with environmental destruction.
- The unattainable standards of "perfection" that get perpetuated within a capitalist society, e.g. pursuit of the "American dream". Activist and queer communities often apply this exact same mentality to setting new standards of what it means to be "radical" - like that a radical person should never feel jealous, never mess up etc.
- Fixation on notions of "independence" - that we should be able to care for 100% of our own needs, which is just plain impossible, even for able-bodied people.
- Tokenizing people with disabilities (or others) by giving only non-decision making roles, inviting last minute participation after visions have been set, and simply having one or two representatives in a group rather than creating ways to genuinely center people with disabilities.
- Setting goals that assume certain types of physical or mental abilities to achieve them.
- Valuing and celebrating only "external" outcomes, like stopping a uranium mine, and devaluing "internal" outcomes, like addressing power and privilege within an

organization/collective.

- Non-profit workers exaggerating results to keep up with funding bodies expectations. Or doing things to look good to our peers, rather than because our actions will create deeper change.
- Making only superficial changes to make something look good for short-term gain, rather than digging to the root causes.

These ways of working are not only able-ist but also racist, classist and colonial too.

I'm left with a lot more questions and ponderings, rather than answers: how do activist and queer groups change cultures of over-work? How do we pay attention to our bodies and create workspaces that care for our bodies? How do we shift what we value to include feminist and disability positive concepts of work? How do movements place people with disabilities at the center instead of at the margins, particularly those who are also people of color, Indigenous, working class, women, queers, trans and gender variant folks and survivors? How do we leverage the gifts that come from the participation of people with non-normative bodies and minds? How can we follow the lead of women of color feminism and embrace the intersections of issues and oppressions? How do we balance striving to do our best with giving up capitalist-influenced definitions of "perfection"? And how do we do all of this whilst working within an urgent context?

This is a big list that I could work on for my whole life. Considering I have been struggling with my changed abilities and my sense of myself as a "valuable" person, today I am going to try to value myself just for being me. That doesn't mean giving up. It means freeing-up all the energy that goes into questioning my worth as a human being - that shit is time-consuming and so draining! It means being able to use that freed-up energy to have a more harmonious relationship with my body and get on with creating change with my communities. And I'm not going to beat myself up if I can't do that "perfectly". In fact, I'm going to celebrate imperfection right now by ending this article perfectly incomplete.

Anna Hamilton

invisibly ill

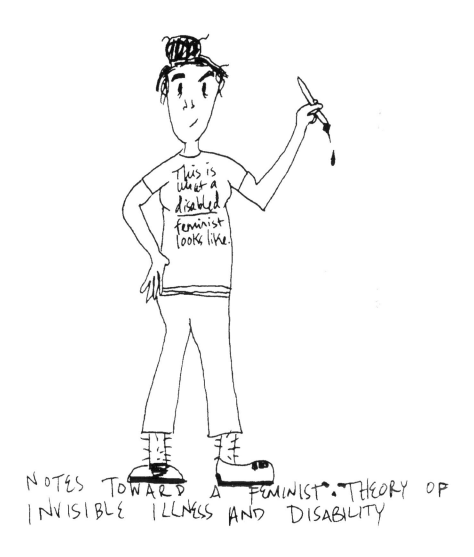

NOTES TOWARD A FEMINIST THEORY OF INVISIBLE ILLNESS AND DISABILITY

A GOOD PLACE TO START...

... WOULD BE THE FOLLOWING ASSERTION...

I have

Fibromyalgia.

IT IS A SYNDROME OF UNKNOWN ORIGIN, CHARACTERIZED BY PHYSICAL PAIN, EXTREME FATIGUE—

AND SO MUCH MORE!

BECAUSE SO MUCH OF MY LIFE FOR THE PAST TWO YEARS HAS BEEN COMPOSED OF DEALING WITH THIS ILLNESS (AFTER GOING FOR 10 MONTHS WITHOUT A DIAGNOSIS, AND THEN A MISDIAGNOSIS; AND THEN BEING TOLD THAT IT WAS PROBABLY "PSYCHOSOMATIC," WHATEVER THE FUCK THAT MEANS; AND THEN FINALLY GETTING AN ACCURATE DIAGNOSIS, NEVER MIND THE CONTINUED DISBELIEF FROM "HEALTHY" PEOPLE, AND THE RESULTING DEPRESSION / "AM I NUTS?!" SELF-FLAGELLATION)... I HAVE DECIDED TO ATTEMPT TO FORMULATE SOMETHING RESEMBLING A FEMINIST THEORETICAL PERSPECTIVE ON "INVISIBLE" ILLNESS.

NOT MANY PEOPLE BELIEVE ME WHEN I TELL THEM THAT I HAVE A DISABILITY!

I FIGURED THAT IT WOULD BE A GOOD IDEA TO DO THIS USING A "NONTRADITIONAL" FORM, AS FIBRO IS NOT A "TRADITIONAL" ILLNESS; AT LEAST, IT'S NOT COMMONLY THOUGHT OF AS A "TRADITIONAL" AILMENT.

MY QUESTIONS ARE THE FOLLOWING:

≥ WHAT ARE SOME OF THE OBSTACLES TO CREATING A THEORY (OR THEORIES) ON EXPERIENCES OF INVISIBLE ILLNESS / DISABILITY?

≥ HOW CAN FEMINIST THEORY HELP?

≥ WHAT WILL IT TAKE TO THEORIZE INVISIBLE ILLNESS, ANYWAY?

≥ WHAT IS AT STAKE, PARTICULARLY WHERE THE BODY IS CONCERNED?

★ I HOPE TO AT LEAST MAKE SOME PROGRESS IN ANSWERING THEM.

DIFFICULTIES! (OR, IMPEDIMENTS TO THE COMPLETION OF THIS PROJECT.)

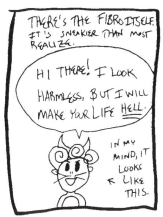

THERE'S THE FIBRO ITSELF. IT IS SNEAKIER THAN MOST REALIZE.

HI THERE! I LOOK HARMLESS, BUT I WILL MAKE YOUR LIFE HELL.

IN MY MIND, IT LOOKS ← LIKE THIS.

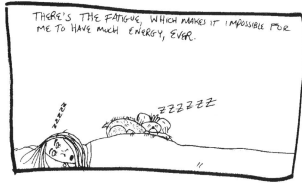

THERE'S THE FATIGUE, WHICH MAKES IT IMPOSSIBLE FOR ME TO HAVE MUCH ENERGY, EVER.

ZZZZZ   ZZZZZZ

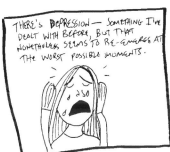

THERE'S DEPRESSION — SOMETHING I'VE DEALT WITH BEFORE, BUT THAT NONETHELESS SEEMS TO RE-EMERGE AT THE WORST POSSIBLE MOMENTS.

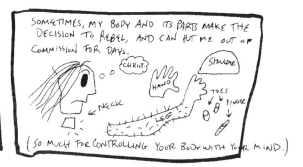

SOMETIMES, MY BODY AND ITS PARTS MAKE THE DECISION TO REBEL, AND CAN PUT ME OUT OF COMMISSION FOR DAYS.

CHRIST   SHOULDER   HAND   ← NECK   LEG   TOES   FINGER

(SO MUCH FOR CONTROLLING YOUR BODY WITH YOUR MIND.)

THERE'S ALSO THE MATTER OF INTENSE PAIN; SOMETIMES, I AM IN SO MUCH PAIN THAT I CAN'T DO ANYTHING.

...EVEN SOMETHING SO "SIMPLE" AS DRAWING.

DIFFICULTIES, PART DEUX

THE QUESTION THAT'S PLAGUED ME FOR A NUMBER OF YEARS...

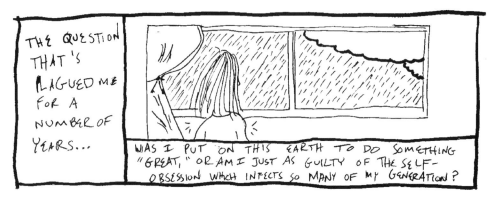

WAS I PUT ON THIS EARTH TO DO SOMETHING "GREAT," OR AM I JUST AS GUILTY OF THE SELF-OBSESSION WHICH INFECTS SO MANY OF MY GENERATION?

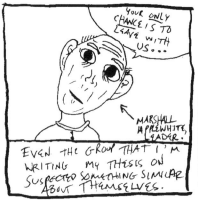

YOUR *ONLY* CHANCE IS TO LEAVE WITH US...

MARSHALL HAPREWHITE, LEADER.

EVEN THE GROUP THAT I'M WRITING MY THESIS ON SUSPECTED SOMETHING SIMILAR ABOUT THEMSELVES.

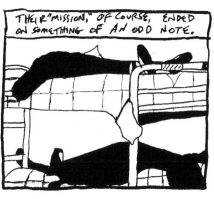

THEIR "MISSION," OF COURSE, ENDED ON SOMETHING OF AN ODD NOTE.

BODIES FOUND IN THEIR MANSION...

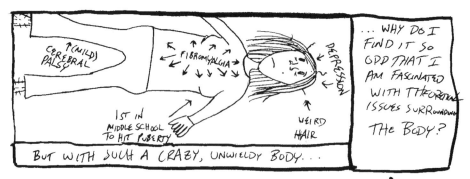

CP (MILD) CEREBRAL PALSY

FIBROMYALGIA

DEPRESSION

1ST IN MIDDLE SCHOOL TO HIT PUBERTY

WEIRD HAIR

BUT WITH SUCH A CRAZY, UNWIELDY BODY...

... WHY DO I FIND IT SO ODD THAT I AM FASCINATED WITH THEORETICAL ISSUES SURROUNDING THE BODY?

I ALSO HAVE MY OWN ISSUES WITH TEXT, AS YOU CAN SEE.

"POSITIVE ATTITUDE" (... IS A BUNCH OF CRAP.)

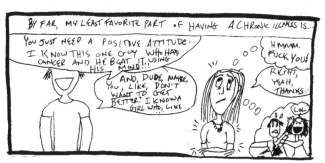

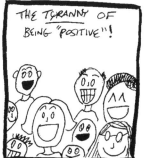

THE TYRANNY OF BEING "POSITIVE"!

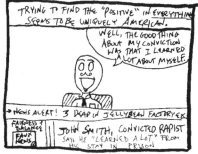

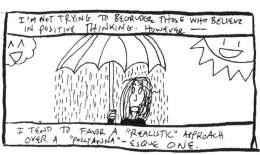

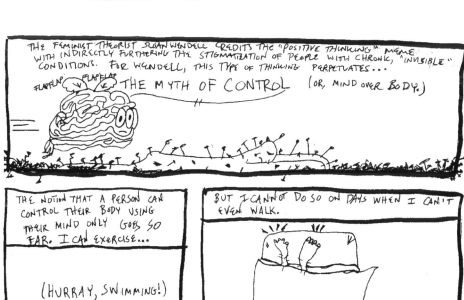

SOME PEOPLE (WHO HAPPEN TO HAVE THE MONEY AND TIME TO DO SO) DEDICATE LARGE PORTIONS OF THEIR LIVES TO "STAYING HEALTHY," ALBEIT IN A SOMEWHAT OVER-THE-TOP MANNER. SOME METHODS OF "HEALTHFUL LIVING" INCLUDE:

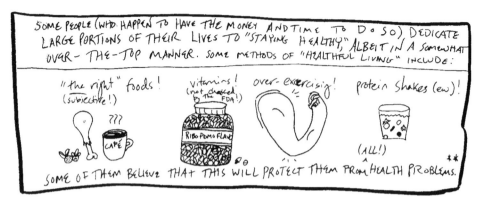

"the right" foods! (subjective!) ??? CAFE

vitamins! (not checked by the FDA!) RIBO POMO FLAVS

over-exercising!

protein shakes (ew)!

(ALL!) **

SOME OF THEM BELIEVE THAT THIS WILL PROTECT THEM FROM HEALTH PROBLEMS.

"HEALTHY" PEOPLE, HOWEVER, ALSO GET SICK AND DIE — JUST LIKE THE REST OF US.

I DON'T GET IT! HE RAN FIVE MILES EVERY DAY.

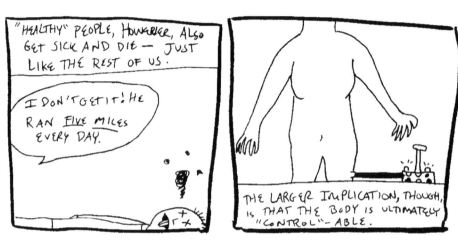

THE LARGER IMPLICATION, THOUGH, IS THAT THE BODY IS ULTIMATELY "CONTROL"-ABLE.

...AND IF YOU CAN'T CONTROL YOUR BODY, YOU HAVE FAILED.

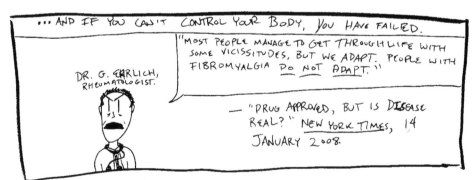

DR. G. EHRLICH, RHEUMATOLOGIST.

"MOST PEOPLE MANAGE TO GET THROUGH LIFE WITH SOME VICISSITUDES, BUT WE ADAPT. PEOPLE WITH FIBROMYALGIA DO NOT ADAPT."

— "DRUG APPROVED, BUT IS DISEASE REAL?" NEW YORK TIMES, 14 JANUARY 2008.

** THIS DEDICATION, IN AND OF ITSELF, IS NOT PROBLEMATIC; IT'S WHEN THOSE WHO PRACTICE IT START TO INSIST THAT THE SAME DEDICATION TO "HEALTH," PRACTICED BY ALL PEOPLE (NO MATTER WHAT THEIR LIMITATIONS), CAN MAGICALLY "CURE" ALL ISSUES, THAT IT BECOMES CREEPY AND PATRONIZING.

INVISIBLE ILLNESS FALLACIES: "HEALTHY" PEOPLE SAY THE DARNDEST THINGS!

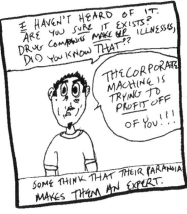

I HAVEN'T HEARD OF IT. ARE YOU SURE IT EXISTS? DRUG COMPANIES MAKE UP ILLNESSES, DID YOU KNOW THAT??

THE CORPORATE MACHINE IS TRYING TO PROFIT OFF OF YOU!!!

SOME THINK THAT THEIR PARANOIA MAKES THEM AN EXPERT.

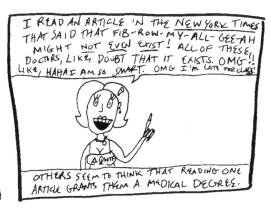

I READ AN ARTICLE IN THE NEW YORK TIMES THAT SAID THAT FIB-ROW-MY-ALL-GEE-AH MIGHT NOT EVEN EXIST! ALL OF THESE DOCTORS, LIKE, DOUBT THAT IT EXISTS. OMG!! LIKE, HAHA I AM SO SMART. OMG I'M LATE FOR CLASS!

OTHERS SEEM TO THINK THAT READING ONE ARTICLE GRANTS THEM A MEDICAL DEGREE.

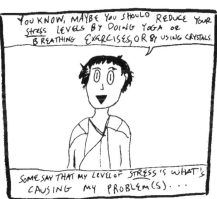

YOU KNOW, MAYBE YOU SHOULD REDUCE YOUR STRESS LEVELS BY DOING YOGA OR BREATHING EXERCISES, OR BY USING CRYSTALS.

SOME SAY THAT MY LEVEL OF STRESS IS WHAT'S CAUSING MY PROBLEM(S) . . .

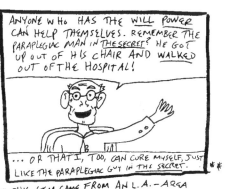

ANYONE WHO HAS THE WILL POWER CAN HELP THEMSELVES. REMEMBER THE PARAPLEGIC MAN IN THE SECRET? HE GOT UP OUT OF HIS CHAIR AND WALKED OUT OF THE HOSPITAL!

. . . OR THAT I, TOO, CAN CURE MYSELF, JUST LIKE THE PARAPLEGIC GUY IN THE SECRET. **

** THIS GEM CAME FROM AN L.A.—AREA HYPNOTIST WHO HAD COME TO THE U.S. FROM ONE OF THE MOST POVERTY-STRICKEN COUNTRIES IN THE WORLD. ⚐

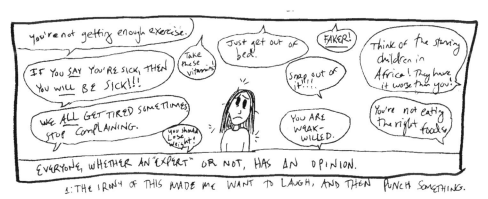

YOU'RE NOT GETTING ENOUGH EXERCISE.

IF YOU SAY YOU'RE SICK, THEN YOU WILL BE SICK!!!

Take these vitamins!

Just get out of bed.

FAKER!

Think of the starving children in Africa! They have it worse than you!

Snap out of it!!!

WE ALL GET TIRED SOMETIMES, STOP COMPLAINING.

You should lose weight!

YOU ARE WEAK-WILLED.

You're not eating the right foods!

EVERYONE, WHETHER AN "EXPERT" OR NOT, HAS AN OPINION.

⚐: THE IRONY OF THIS MADE ME WANT TO LAUGH, AND THEN PUNCH SOMETHING.

PASSING

THE MODERN PERSON WITH AN INVISIBLE DISABILITY IS STUCK IN A CONUNDRUM.

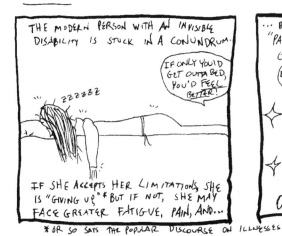

ZZZZZE

IF ONLY YOU'D GET OUTTA BED, YOU'D FEEL BETTER!

IF SHE ACCEPTS HER LIMITATIONS, SHE IS "GIVING UP"* BUT IF NOT, SHE MAY FACE GREATER FATIGUE, PAIN, AND...

... BE NONETHELESS PRESSURED TO "PASS" AS NORMAL; AS NOT ILL OR DISABLED...

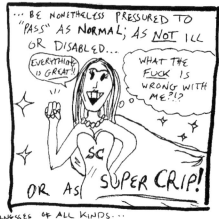

EVERYTHING IS GREAT!!

WHAT THE FUCK IS WRONG WITH ME?!?

SC

OR AS SUPER CRIP!

*OR SO SAYS THE POPULAR DISCOURSE ON ILLNESSES OF ALL KINDS...

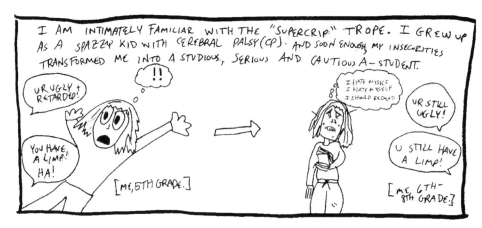

I AM INTIMATELY FAMILIAR WITH THE "SUPERCRIP" TROPE. I GREW UP AS A SPAZZY KID WITH CEREBRAL PALSY (CP). AND SOON ENOUGH, MY INSECURITIES TRANSFORMED ME INTO A STUDIOUS, SERIOUS AND CAUTIOUS A-STUDENT.

!!

UR UGLY + RETARDED!

YOU HAVE A LIMP! HA!

[ME, 5TH GRADE.]

I HATE MYSELF
I HATE MYSELF
I SHOULD BE DEAD

UR STILL UGLY!

U STILL HAVE A LIMP!

[ME, 6TH-8TH GRADE.]

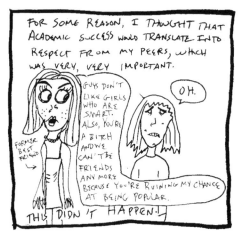

FOR SOME REASON, I THOUGHT THAT ACADEMIC SUCCESS WOULD TRANSLATE INTO RESPECT FROM MY PEERS, WHICH WAS VERY, VERY IMPORTANT.

GUYS DON'T LIKE GIRLS WHO ARE SMART. ALSO, YOU'RE A BITCH AND WE CAN'T BE FRIENDS ANYMORE BECAUSE YOU'RE RUINING MY CHANCE AT BEING POPULAR.

OH.

FORMER BEST FRIEND

THIS DIDN'T HAPPEN.

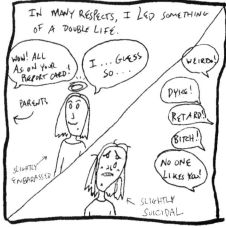

IN MANY RESPECTS, I LED SOMETHING OF A DOUBLE LIFE.

WOW! ALL As ON YOUR REPORT CARD!

I... GUESS SO...

PARENTS

SLIGHTLY EMBARASSED

WEIRDO!

DYKE!

RETARD!

BITCH!

NO ONE LIKES YOU!

SLIGHTLY SUICIDAL

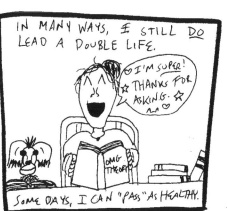

IN MANY WAYS, I STILL DO LEAD A DOUBLE LIFE.

♥ I'M SUPER! ☆ THANKS FOR ASKING. ☆

SOME DAYS, I CAN "PASS" AS HEALTHY.

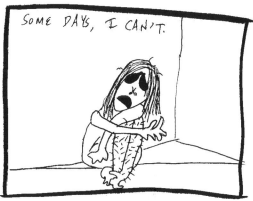

SOME DAYS, I CAN'T.

ELAINE SCARRY, IN HER SEMINAL WORK THE BODY IN PAIN, NOTES THAT "TO HAVE PAIN IS TO HAVE CERTAINTY; TO HEAR ABOUT PAIN IS TO HAVE DOUBT."*

THE NATURE OF A CONDITION SUCH AS FIBROMYALGIA — WHERE SOME WHO HAVE IT CAN "INHABIT" DUAL WORLDS — MAKES THE DISPARITY¹ QUITE PRONOUNCED.

[AND HAVE]

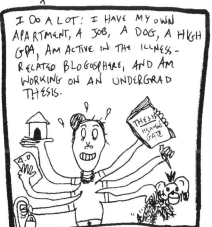

I DO A LOT: I HAVE MY OWN APARTMENT, A JOB, A DOG, A HIGH GPA, AM ACTIVE IN THE ILLNESS-RELATED BLOGOSPHERE, AND AM WORKING ON AN UNDERGRAD THESIS.

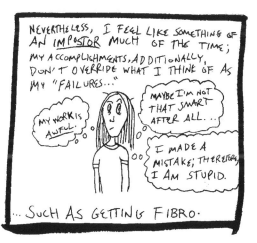

NEVERTHELESS, I FEEL LIKE SOMETHING OF AN IMPOSTOR MUCH OF THE TIME; MY ACCOMPLISHMENTS, ADDITIONALLY, DON'T OVERRIDE WHAT I THINK OF AS MY "FAILURES..."

MY WORK IS AWFUL.

MAYBE I'M NOT THAT SMART AFTER ALL...

I MADE A MISTAKE; THEREFORE, I AM STUPID.

... SUCH AS GETTING FIBRO.

* SCARRY 13.

1: I MEAN THE DISPARITY BETWEEN PAIN-RELATED CERTAINTY AND DOUBT; I RAN OUT OF SPACE IN THIS PANEL. OOPS.

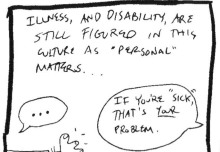

ILLNESS, AND DISABILITY, ARE STILL FIGURED IN THIS CULTURE AS "PERSONAL" MATTERS...

...

IF YOU'RE "SICK," THAT'S YOUR PROBLEM.

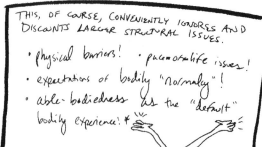

THIS, OF COURSE, CONVENIENTLY IGNORES AND DISCOUNTS LARGER STRUCTURAL ISSUES.

- physical barriers!   • pace-of-life issues!
- expectations of bodily "normalcy"!
- able-bodiedness as the "default" bodily experience! *

WITH THE ADVENT OF NEW-AGE THINKING AND THE IDEA THAT "YOU CREATE YOUR OWN REALITY," (AMONG OTHER THINGS), CHRONIC, DISABLING HEALTH CONDITIONS ARE FIGURED AS SOMEHOW CONTROL-ABLE. THE ATTITUDES AGAINST THOSE WITH THESE CONDITIONS ARE, THEREFORE, DE-POLITICIZED, INSTEAD OF SEEN AS SYMPTOMATIC OF ANY LARGER BIASES AGAINST THOSE WITH NON-VISIBLE, CHRONIC, AND DISABLING CONDITIONS.

REMEMBER, YOU CREATE YOUR OWN REALITY. THIS IS HARD TO ACCEPT, BUT IT IS THE BLAH BLAH...

MY "REALITY" DOES NOT INCLUDE THIS BLAME-Y BULLSHIT!!

(SOME DAYS, WE HAVE THE ENERGY TO FIGHT BACK.)

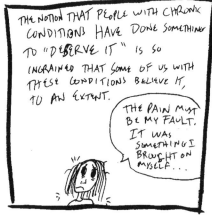

THE NOTION THAT PEOPLE WITH CHRONIC CONDITIONS HAVE DONE SOMETHING TO "DESERVE IT" IS SO INGRAINED THAT SOME OF US WITH THESE CONDITIONS BELIEVE IT, TO AN EXTENT.

THE PAIN MUST BE MY FAULT. IT WAS SOMETHING I BROUGHT ON MYSELF...

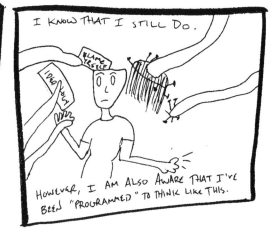

I KNOW THAT I STILL DO.

HOWEVER, I AM ALSO AWARE THAT I'VE BEEN "PROGRAMMED" TO THINK LIKE THIS.

1: "THE SECRET," 2006.
* MCRUER 1.

FUN WITH STIGMA (AND [IN]VISIBILITY)

THERE IS STILL A LARGE AMOUNT OF STIGMA SURROUNDING CHRONIC, "INVISIBLE" ILLNESSES / DISABILITIES, AND WHICH SURROUNDS THOSE WHO LIVE WITH THESE CONDITIONS . . .

FUCK.

AS SUSAN WENDELL HAS POINTED OUT, "[P]EOPLE WONDER WHETHER SOMEONE WHOSE DISABILITY IS NOT OBVIOUS IS FAKING OR EXAGGERATING IT; THE TRUSTWORTHINESS OF PEOPLE WHO CLAIM TO BE DISABLED BUT DO NOT LOOK DISABLED IS ALWAYS IN QUESTION" (29).

BUT... YOU'RE TOO YOUNG TO BE DISABLED! YOU COULD BE FAKING IT TO GET SYMPATHY — I CAN'T SEE IT, SO HOW DO I KNOW IT'S REAL!??!

OUR CULTURAL CONCEPTIONS OF DISABILITY RELY SO MUCH ON THE VISUAL SIGNS OF "DISABILITY", AND PEOPLE WHOSE DISABILITIES ARE NOT APPARENT GO AGAINST THIS VERY INGRAINED TROPE.

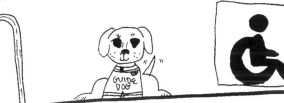

ON SOME LEVEL, THIS "NEW" FORM OF DISABILITY IS UNDERSTANDABLY CONFUSING TO ABLE-BODIED FOLKS.

OH, WE'RE ALL "DISABLED" IN SOME WAY. SUCK IT UP.

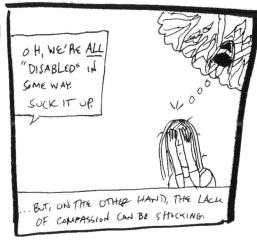

...BUT, ON THE OTHER HAND, THE LACK OF COMPASSION CAN BE SHOCKING.

EVERYBODY LOVES TALKING ABOUT CLASS!

WHEN I WAS A KID, MY PARENTS (TO THEIR CREDIT) DID NOT ENCOURAGE ME TO THINK OF MYSELF AS "DISABLED," EVEN WITH MY C.P.

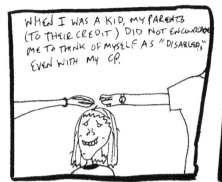

MOST OF THE TIME, THIS WORKED.

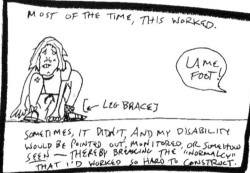

[← LEG BRACE]

LAME FOOT!

SOMETIMES, IT DIDN'T, AND MY DISABILITY WOULD BE POINTED OUT, MONITORED, OR SOMEHOW SEEN — THEREBY BREAKING THE "NORMALCY" THAT I'D WORKED SO HARD TO CONSTRUCT.

SINCE BEING DIAGNOSED WITH FIBRO, I AM NO LONGER AS RELUCTANT TO IDENTIFY MYSELF AS DISABLED, OR AS A PERSON WITH A DISABILITY; THIS IS MOSTLY BECAUSE THE FIBRO *DOES* DIS-ABLE ME QUITE FREQUENTLY, AND I AM IN NEAR-CONSTANT PHYSICAL PAIN.

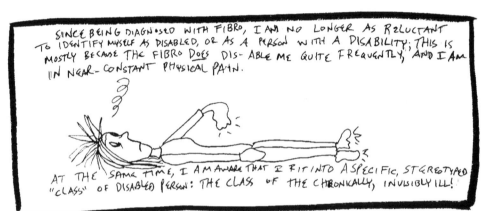

AT THE SAME TIME, I AM AWARE THAT I FIT INTO A SPECIFIC, STEREOTYPED "CLASS" OF DISABLED PERSON: THE CLASS OF THE CHRONICALLY, INVISIBLY ILL!

THE STEREOTYPE OF THE CHRONICALLY AND INVISIBLY ILL LOOKS SOMETHING LIKE THE FOLLOWING:

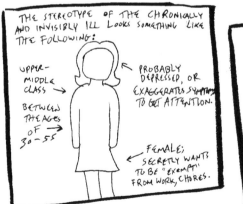

UPPER-MIDDLE CLASS →

BETWEEN THE AGES OF → 30-55

← PROBABLY DEPRESSED, OR EXAGGERATES SYMPTOMS TO GET ATTENTION.

← FEMALE; SECRETLY WANTS TO BE "EXEMPT" FROM WORK, CHORES.

THE PROBLEM WITH THESE STEREOTYPES IS THAT THEY CONTRIBUTE TO MISUNDERSTANDINGS OF WHAT IS, IN ACTUALITY, A COMPLICATED CONDITION.

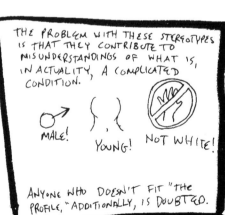

MALE!

YOUNG!

NOT WHITE!

ANYONE WHO DOESN'T FIT "THE PROFILE," ADDITIONALLY, IS DOUBTED.

HOW CAN FEMINIST THEORY HELP (AND WHY)?

ACCORDING TO BOTH SUSAN WENDELL AND JOURNALIST PAULA KAMEN, INVISIBLE ILLNESS IS DEFINITELY A FEMINIST ISSUE.

THIS IS NOT ONLY BECAUSE THE SOCIAL MEANINGS + STEREOTYPES SURROUNDING INVISIBLE ILLNESS ARE COMMONLY THOUGHT OF AS "FEMINIZED"* BUT ALSO BECAUSE THE FEMINIST MOVEMENT STILL HOLDS ABLEIST BIASES[1]

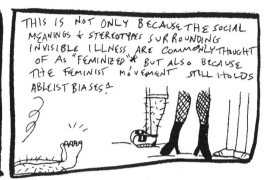

WENDELL CONTENDS THAT "MUCH FEMINIST PRACTICE STILL ASSUMES A CONSISTENTLY ENERGETIC, HIGH-FUNCTIONING BODY AND MIND..." (24)

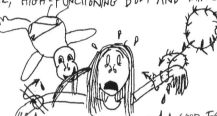

SHE CONTINUES: "THE ACCEPTED IMAGE OF A GOOD FEMINIST STILL INCLUDES... WORK AND FAMILY...AND HAVING PLENTY OF ENERGY LEFT OVER FOR POLITICAL ACTIVITY IN THE EVENINGS OR ON WEEKENDS."[2]

IF THE GOAL OF THE FEMINIST MOVEMENT IS, IN PART, TO COUNTER CULTURAL AND SOCIAL BIASES OF MANY INTERSECTING KINDS, THE ISSUES OF FEMINISTS WITH CHRONIC ILLNESSES MUST BE ADDRESSED.

A FEMINIST THEORY ON INVISIBLE ILLNESS AND DISABILITY WOULD TAKE ON THE STEREOTYPICAL VIEWS OF THESE CONDITIONS AS "FEMALE"; THIS THEORY WOULD ALSO ADDRESS THOSE WHO LIVE WITH THESE CONDITIONS, AND TAKE SUCH AN ADDRESS AS A STARTING POINT FOR WIDER CRITIQUE AND CHANGE.

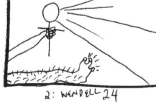

* BARKER 207; KAMEN 161-163
1: WENDELL 24-25

2: WENDELL 24

WHAT'S AT STAKE

OF COURSE, WITH THE INTRODUCTION OF ANY NEW THEORETICAL IDEAS OR PERSPECTIVES, PROBLEMS MAY ARISE.

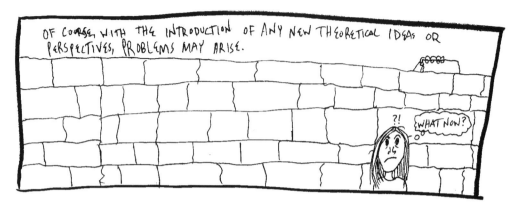

?!
WHAT NOW?

WE MUST TAKE CARE, ADDITIONALLY, IN RECOGNIZING THAT EXPERIENCES WITH INVISIBLE ILLNESS — PARTICULARLY IN A CORPOREAL SENSE — ARE VARIED, AS ARE THE PEOPLE WHO HAVE THESE ILLNESSES.

I'D GIVE YOU A HIGH FIVE, BUT MY HAND HURTS TOO MUCH.

SAME HERE.

AT THE SAME TIME, RECOGNIZING COMMON GROUND IS IMPORTANT.

THOSE WHO HAVE <u>NOT</u> HAD EXPERIENCES WITH LIFE-CHANGING ILLNESS, DISABILITY, OR PAIN MAY ALSO BE RESISTANT TO THE SUBJECTHOOD AND TESTIMONIES OF THE INVISIBLY ILL/ DISABLED.

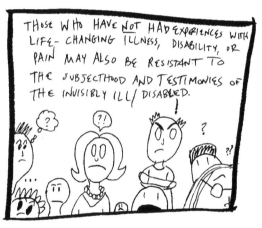

SUSAN WENDELL CONTENDS THAT THOSE WITH INVISIBLE ILLNESSES/DISABILITIES ARE OFTEN PRESSURED TO "PASS" AS NOT ILL, OR TO CONSTANTLY REASSURE THOSE WITHOUT SIMILAR CONDITIONS THAT THEY DO, IN FACT, "CONFORM... TO AN INSPIRING VERSION OF THE PARADIGM OF DISABILITY" (22).

I'M GREAT!

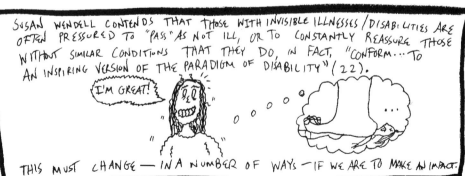

THIS MUST CHANGE — IN A NUMBER OF WAYS — IF WE ARE TO MAKE AN IMPACT.

SOLUTIONS?

OBLIGATORY DISCLAIMER:

DUE TO THE SHORTNESS OF THIS PROJECT, MY SOLUTIONS MAY NOT BE FULLY UN-PROBLEMATIC.

RATHER THAN SIMPLY "RAISING AWARENESS," I MAINTAIN THAT A COMPREHENSIVE THEORY OF INVISIBLE ILLNESS IS NEEDED; THE FIRST STEP IS RECOGNIZING THE IMPORTANCE OF CHALLENGING THE BIASES THAT EXIST, STARTING ON A MICRO-LEVEL. SOME IDEAS INCLUDE...

 BLOGS:

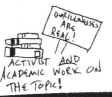 ACTIVIST AND ACADEMIC WORK ON THE TOPIC!

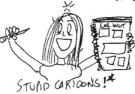 STUPID CARTOONS!*

* OKAY, MAYBE NOT.

PEOPLE WITH THESE ILLNESSES AND CONDITIONS MUST BE WILLING TO "STEP UP" AND SPEAK ABOUT THEIR EXPERIENCES (IN ADDITION TO OTHER THINGS) IN ORDER TO SHIFT THE POWERS THAT BE.

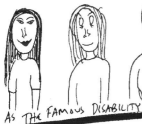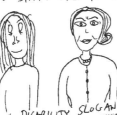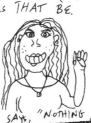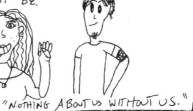

AS THE FAMOUS DISABILITY SLOGAN SAYS, "NOTHING ABOUT US WITHOUT US."

FINALLY, WE MUST BE WILLING TO FORM A THEORY THAT IS OPEN TO SHIFTS, CHANGES, AND COMPLICATIONS. IN HIS BOOK CRIP THEORY, ROBERT MCRUER CONTENDS THAT A "QUEER" THEORY OF DISABILITY COULD "CONTINUOUSLY INVOKE" AND QUESTION "THE INADEQUATE RESOLUTIONS THAT COMPULSORY ABLE-BODIEDNESS AND COMPULSORY HETEROSEXUALITY OFFER US." [1]

THESE CHANGES WILL NOT HAPPEN OVERNIGHT, BUT THEY MUST BE MADE.

1: MCRUER 31.   The end.

mental illness and a herniated disc
a brutal combination

I was born a fighter. I never, ever give up. I am not afraid of very much and nothing really shocks me. I am in my late thirties and I have been "mentally ill" my entire life. Having known no other life, that is the life I've lived. I was mental illness and that was really the end of the story. I had no future and no reason for hope. I had lived in three different group homes. I had been on countless medications that not only did not work, but because of these drugs I was condemned to live with some very terrible side effects. I was such a victim, a thrown away person. The side effects that I experienced as a teenager were both dreadful and hellish and I live with very deep emotional and physical scars because of them to this day.

I have lived with the symptoms of mental illness for all of my life. My life was unfulfilling and my interactions with most everyone I came in contact with were at least in some ways tremendously unhealthy. Due to my symptoms and never having learned how to take care of myself or manage my symptoms, all of my relationships and connections with other people were compromised and decaying in various degrees of dysfunction. I was already more or less alone, isolated and alienated and this was my everyday life.

In 2002, my back was hurting and I could not figure out what was wrong with me. Within a few days I could not walk. These were some of the worst days of my life. I got myself to the emergency room where I was told I had a pulled muscle and was given some muscle relaxers and some painkillers and sent home. I was clearly disabled and unable to care for myself.

I had terrible roommates at the time, being an adult with mental illness who had no job, life, friends or any real support network, social or otherwise. These roommates were dirty, strange and very unhelpful. Over the course of the next few months due to being unable to care for myself and having received almost no help at all from anyone, I shed over 40 pounds, crawled, took taxis to all my appointments and my family while being only a 30 minute drive away, did nothing.

Somehow I had it in me to fight to stay alive throughout this ordeal. My quality of life was already awful before the introduction of the physically and mentally crippling pain that had taken over all aspects of my life. The mental damage that I was now suffering was 1000 times worse than my worst nightmare. I was so afraid that I would never have a life again, even a life as rotten as the one I had. Desperately I wanted help to alleviate the destruction that was happening to me and my life.

By chance, just as this life crisis had begun, I received a package in the mail from a pen pal in Mexico. In this package there was a cassette by a band named Petrograd who were from Luxembourg. I had never listened to Petrograd before and upon putting this tape into my boom box and pressing play I heard the most beautiful and hopeful music, more beautiful and hopeful than any other music I have ever heard in my entire life. I would play this tape again and again and again, as I knew my life as I knew it was over and I felt something spiritual happening to me when I listened to Petrograd. This music gave me endless hope and it does to this day. Hope was all that I had and I did not have much else and the impact that this music had on my life and my survival in my darkest of days is immeasurable.

So I took countless taxis back and forth to the chiropractor, the physical therapist, the primary care physician, the spine specialist and for more emergency room visits. Each and every time I was told that I had a pulled muscle. At this point I was months into being incapacitated and I was doing everything I could to help myself and I hit a brick wall at every turn, a brick wall that usually took money from me. I was miserable, sick and incapacitated with no hope for an end in sight. I wanted to die.

Unfortunately those people out there that most of us have in our lives, namely friends, had more or less disappeared from my life. There were a few people who visited once, a couple who visited twice and then silence. No one wanted to spend time with a physically and mentally ill man. It would have been helpful if someone would have assisted me but there was no one there. Friends and family alike were just not there and unwilling to do much of anything. I needed real help. I needed friends. I needed my family. But there was only me, mentally ill, physically incapacitated, broke, unable to take care of myself, doomed to suffer and die hopeless and in pain.

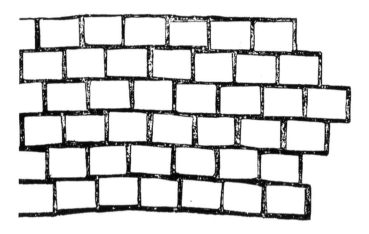

My mental state was at a dangerous place. I was already ill and I had no skills, no money, nothing to do, no hope, no options and I was in hell. I can remember the extremes of the sickness I was experiencing. My mind and my thoughts were frighteningly out of control. I was facing the end of who I was and I was doomed. I continued to go back and forth to the chiropractor, the physical therapist and the primary care physician while clearly in extreme physical pain. My body was contorted and rigid and I was dragging myself around, barely. I went to these health providers for them to help me and they did nothing. The one thing they did do was throw me away like a piece of garbage and that is what I was, and that is what I became. I was confused, I had nothing and life was becoming meaningless.

This devastating injury of mine began around the beginning of March 2002. The rental agreement for the apartment where I was living was going to be up at the end of August and I needed to find a new place to live. This is an extremely hard thing to do when you are clearly incapacitated, have no job, do nothing all day, have no real money and basically are the worst possible candidate to move into someone else's apartment ever. Why would anyone in their right mind allow me, at that point in time, to move into their place? I was an absolute disaster. I needed serious medical care and medical intervention yet no matter how hard I tried to get help and treatment, I failed again and again and again.

Either way, I was forced to answer personal ads and go meet people and look at rooms. I took public transportation to achieve this. How ridiculous do you think it was to see this young man dragging himself around, absolutely desperate and incapacitated, going to meet people with rooms available? I was obviously a terrible candidate and of course none of these people offered me a room. In fact they would have had to have serious issues if they thought that I was going to work out for them.

Up until this point my family continued to not help me. This is probably due firstly to my mental health issues and secondly the fact that my aunt had been dying and then died and they were busy. However my family could have helped alleviate my suffering and up until this point they had chosen not to. As the days crept closer to when I would have to be out of my apartment, I grew increasingly nervous and apprehensive and became sicker and sicker.

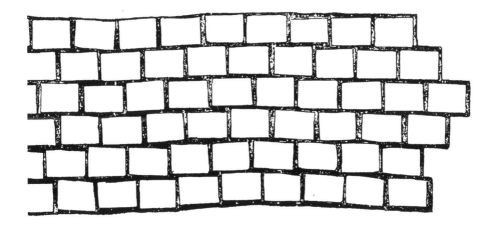

With my mental health in tatters, being destitute and broke and alone and desperate was bad enough. Unfortunately, the constant onslaught of crippling pain had become fused with the poor mental health and I was now a completely broken person. Mental illness and herniated discs are each on their own absolutely devastating and life destroying, yet the miserable and torturous combination of both horrendous conditions had left me an empty shell of person. It was as if I had survived a bomb blast and I was stuck under a mountain of rubble. I was breathing but without a miracle, and a miracle soon, all I would be is breathing and at some point dead.

Within ten days of having nowhere to live, my parents came and took me to see their primary care physician. He took one look at me and said he was pretty sure I had a herniated disc and I needed an MRI right away. The MRI was scheduled within a few days and the results showed a severally herniated L4/L5 disc. I was physically destroyed and the prospect of life had ended. The suffering was beyond anything I have ever known. My parents begrudgingly allowed me to move into their home so I could have surgery and get back on my feet.

During this experience I had endured a lot of mistreatment from the mouths of people who should have known better. My life was already pathetic before a herniated disc destroyed what was left of it and people for some reason found me unapproachable. Perhaps having been so physically damaged people didn't know what to do, yet my level of mental sickness made it impossible for people to be around me. I still question why people were so unkind to me. Perhaps I made it difficult for people to be in my presence. Perhaps I was so sick that my memory was skewed. Regardless of the specifics, I am fully aware that people were not nice to me. I still know those people today. Having a back injury and a mental health condition at the same time is grounds for abuse for a lot of people. I suppose as they are both invisible injuries and sicknesses, and that people's empathy goes out the door when dealing with situations where you can't see what the issue is. The same applied to my circumstances

At the very end of August, having my body relentlessly riddled with shooting pain and with my nerves causing such disruptive sensations in my legs; I was more or less relegated to my bedroom. My bedroom was my only safe place to be yet the only place in my room that would I spend my time was lying on my mattress. After so many months of being unable to properly care for myself, my body, my clothes and my bed had become dirtier than I would have liked. I was sleeping on a mattress without any sheets in the dead of summer without any air conditioning. Yeah, it smelled terrible. That was where I found myself, sitting alone, isolated, terrified about my future, terrified about my life and surrounded by a most unpleasant smell that I could do nothing about. I remember sitting on the mattress and having a thought. Well, I am not sure if it was just a thought or if I actually said it out loud. To this day I have no idea which it was: in my thoughts or spoken aloud from my mouth. The words or thoughts however, I distinctly recall: "If you make it out of this in one piece then you need to change your life for the better."

On September 1st 2002, I moved to my parent's home. I had surgery on my lower back at the end of October. I had my mobility back and a bit of hope for a future. My parents and I clashed often and it was not pretty however as awful that it was that they left me to rot and suffer; they also for whatever reason rescued me from my own demise. I do thank them for this.

I have had two more disc herniations and subsequent operations on the L4/L5 since my first time in 2002, once in 2007 and once in 2009. I am an old pro.

Here it is 2011, I am mentally healthy. I have gone to school and I work as a peer mental health counselor at the same hospital where I have had my surgeries. My success is a result of my suffering. It is beautiful. Now that I've had three recurrent disc herniations I have finally gotten my act together and I am taking care of myself. I have lost over 60 pounds and I do my stretches and go for therapeutic walks, therapeutic both mentally and physically, almost everyday. I am going to be OK and I am OK.

I am a success, a success that nobody in 2002 believed in so take a good look at me now. I have come full circle. I have become self-actualized and I like me. I would not be who I am today without all of my experiences including all of the terrible things I have been through, yet I exist. Not only do I exist, I am thriving because of all of this. I would not change a thing about my past.

I am a success now and I will be a success in the future directly because I know what hell is. Hell has an address and I know there is an open invitation for me to visit. I may end up stopping by at some point in the future but there is no way that I am moving in ever again.

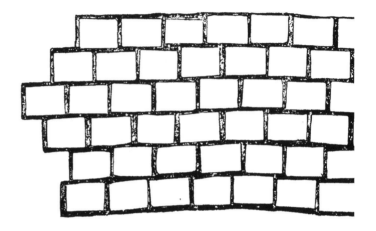

Noemi Martinez

sin mas

Gloria,
We all want to take a part (of) you, swallow
it, say you were
here, you were ours. You are.
I see fotos of you & it's like I knew you.
Some crazy loca queer Chicana on Chicana crush
que no sé ni de que o de que viene.

my only regrets   are with those   who have passed
You were 34 when I was born
Now that age

We follow your words

When I learned it was diabetes that took you in your sleep
que se robo tus palabras que no habías escrito
I think about the insulin shots mi mami tiene aqui
in the refrigerator.
I think of my hermana's unchecked sugar levels
& a mother's worry
I began to see how we ate, what we ate, what poisons come,
hurt our espíritu, our alma, llevando pedacitos

When they let us nonacademic common folks see those boxes
held within walls, pedazos de ti,
will I find recetas de nopalitos
clippings de comida que deberíamos comer?

How else can we stop the poisons that
infiltrate our beings, our souls, it's constant
if not the food, simply the being.

My teacher, my guide, i
wear your words
on my side, on my chest
en un bulto, aqui as if i knew you

I see fotos, 2002, you in San Antonio.
¿Porque no estaba allí?
Workshop for queer writers ¿Porque no estaba allí?
Is this blasphemy, saying I am not the bridge

Sometimes what we consume it what kills us.
Maybe the violence of our eating
lives in our cells

Why do these poisons come
that eat away our writing mothers?

También I search your writing, your words
in dealing with this pain, de que no se habla
because admitting pain is a luxury
las del valle cannot afford.
I ask my professor friends here & there to email & scan
articles & papers for me about your writing,
your pain
the dark side of your selves-
being a nonacademic, they are not available to me
You would get a kick out of that.

Sin Mas, Esperando
Noemí

claire barrera

resisting erasure

The day after I was sexually assaulted, I stood before a painting
by Frida Khalo in the Dolores Olmeda museum on the parched
outskirts of D.F., Mexico. I had taken the metro out and walked
around the sprawling grounds which were full of agave, peacocks
and the Xoloitzcuintli, an ancient breed of hairless dogs Khalo
loved. I paced through the many rooms of the hacienda which
were full of precolonial art and the paintings of Diego Rivera.
Finally, I arrived at a small room beyond a courtyard where
the painting "Henry Ford Hospital, 1932" is housed. It is a self
portrait by Khalo painted after a miscarriage she had at Henry
Ford Hospital, due to a pelvic injury she sustained in a bus crash
years before. She lies in a hospital bed, blood pooling beneath
her, while three umbelical chords lead to a fetus, a pink plaster
figure and a snail, respectively. The painted Frida is crying, and
an orchid, a steely machine and her shattered pelvis lie on the
ground beside her bed.

I was alone in the room and it was quiet. I bent to read the
title and explanation hung beside the painting. I recall the
description telling of the miscarriage, and the recurring theme
of loss surrounding Kahlo's work regarding her inability to
have children. This description also ventured that Kahlo had
exaggerated her desire to have children and her sense of loss for
artistic purposes, and that really she had not wanted a child so
badly as she wanted dramatic subject matter for her paintings.

Just like that, the author had erased Khalo's self-definition in
this incredible work of art. Using his or her priviledge as an art
curator, this person had effortlessly deleted the story of her
pain and replaced it with his/her own "educated" interpretation.
Susan Greenhalgh aptly describes this replacement when she
recounts her own experience of a male doctor disregarding her
personal narrative of her illness. Like Greenhalgh's, Khalo's
"own version of her bodily past had been erased," the author's
"substituted for it" (Greenhalgh 69).

Just that morning, I had stood at the window of my hostel in D.F. for almost 5 hours watching for my assaulter. Hoping he would not appear again to wait for me in the plaza below, scanning the crowds of tourists and vendors and lovers and punks and shoppers and business men for his face. My heart beat so fast against my ribs. I was already plagued with the doubt and self-blame all survivors of trauma experience. Standing before Khalo's art, I identified so strongly with the message of pain and loss in Khalo's painting. And as I saw the author of the painting's description nullify Khalo's message, I too felt my truth about my experience begin to be undermined, and to disappear.

I remember this Brazillian chiropractor practicing in San Francisco once told me, "Latinas are usually not very flexible." He was surprised by my dancer body's ability to move so easily, in spite of the pain and tightness of my muscles.

I thought how, when you carry a great many people's histories on your bones; including but not limited to rape, torture, exploitation, which not only happened to you but your sister and her daughter and her daughters' friend, and also your land, and you are carrying your future strapped tightly to your chest, sucking its thumb, and you are also carrying your gifts of loving and healing, at times bending over backwards to provide them - well yes, your tendons and ligaments may have tightened some. When you have worked twice, three times as hard to carve out a space in the world and it probably included evenings and weekends, you are bound to be sore and inflexible.

In her book of poetry and pensamientos, "Loving in the War Year", queer and Chicana author Cherie Moraga writes,

> "Sometimes I feel my back will break from the
> pressure I feel to speak for others. A friend told
> me once how no wonder I had called the first
> book I co-edited (with Gloria Anzaldua) "This
> Bridge Called My Back". You have chronic back
> trouble, she says. Funny, I never considered
> this most obvious connection, all along my back
> giving me constant pain." (Moraga v)

Moraga is saying her need to voice the story of her people's identity is a great weight she carries, causing real pain to her body.

Being a womyn, and a womyn of color, and a queer womyn of color means experiencing an acute sense of invisibility and for Moraga and many others, there is a need to speak out against this invisibility. Further, having these identities means carrying the weight of our mutual and often painful history on our backs every day. What ailment more literal than chronic back pain? It is a pain caused by a burden too heavy to be carried without trauma to our spines. Further, it is an ailment as invisible as we are forced to be in this world. It was not until I began to experience more severe back pain that I began to meet so many others like myself, usually womyn, often queer womyn or womyn of color (or both), who suffered this illness themselves. Talking with those I have met, I recognized our common experiences. Like Cherie Moraga, I had a realization about the direct connection between my pain and my identity.

I already live in a world in which I have fought to be seen, and seen on my own terms. People belonging to groups oppressed by the dominant culture have always been in danger of erasure. Our languages, ways of healing, our food, our stories: all continue to be methodically scratched off the surface of the earth. Yet it is not just our cultures that are threatened with disappearance. The very ways we choose to identify are denied us.

In my father's family, we have slowly lost our connections to our Mexican ancestry. My father and his siblings were discouraged from speaking Spanish, both at home by their parents and at school. Familial ties in Mexico were slowly cut, until no one ever crossed the border anymore to visit the aunts and uncles on the other side. As he grew older, my father strove to assimilate with white American culture as best he could, shedding his cultural past in an attempt to find a better future. Some of it cannot be retrieved.

Growing up, I always felt the void where my family's history used to be. It was like a cold wind blowing in the emptiness behind me, raising the hairs on my neck. Some of our story had been erased by the hands of hegemony. It has been challenging to assert my existence and identity in the present, in spite of what was lost in the past. For so long I did not even have names by which to call myself, those names that I have now- queer, Xicana, among others. The culture around me was telling that my experience did not or should not exist. That I am invisible. I carry the trauma of those times I was given this message, and it weighs me down.

For myself and for most others, chronic pain has physical causes and is a real illness. It can also be a manifestation of emotional and psychological trauma and a sense of invisibility. It serves to aggravate these problems. Chickasaw poet and novelist Linda Hogan recounts in her memoir how she lost her ability to dream due to fibromyalgia she developed. As an "ancient measure" of herself, Hogan had always counted on her ability to dream and her ability to connect with the holy through her dreams. Yet she lost this fundamental ability when she developed chronic pain. She writes,

> "The inner story slipped away from me, my
> self was dismantled, unbuilt... My faith in the
> body and its vitality was lost, and losing faith
> in the body a person inhabits and has been in
> good relationship with is frightening... In pain
> there is the unmaking of a person, an identity, a
> world." (Hogan 132)

Hogan's pain reflected a long history of trauma both she and her people had suffered. In a sense, the pain dug this trauma to the surface, worrying it like a person worries a scab until it bleeds, causing a fresh wound. Hogan's pain highlighted her past suffering, at the same time it caused her new injury by destroying the ways she had formerly stayed connected to her identity and given it voice in the world.

Having chronic pain does not garner the visibility and support one may wish and long for. On the contrary, in my experience it has provided oppressive systems with a new way to negate me. As it did for Hogan, this negation has come from the loss of the means by which I affirm and express my identities. I have also experienced it through the ways I have been treated by anyone from doctors, to family and friends, to strangers on the street. Certainly, my attempts at accessing patriarchal western medical care led me to many hurtful and demeaning experiences.

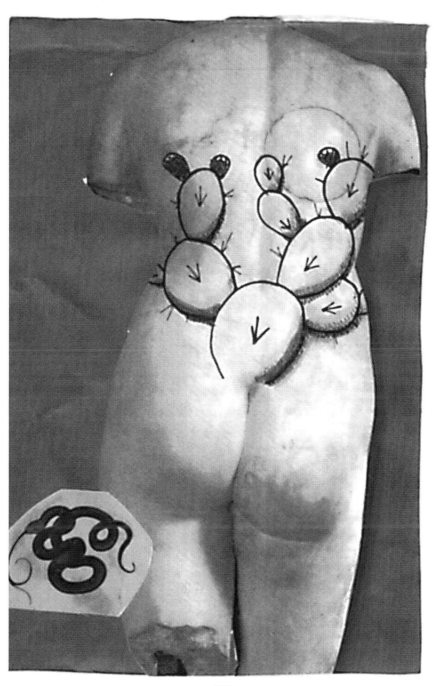

A few years after I was assaulted, my pain had reached a high point. I went to see a physiatrist (a musculoskeletal expert) about my chronic back pain. It seemed like he was the billionth doctor I had been to in the last few years. None of them had the explanation as to why I was in so much pain and why none of their treatments where helping. I had just started recieving insurance with Kaiser Permanente and it had taken me three months of phone calls and self-advocacy to get to this appointment. I came armed with a list of the medications I was on, therapies I'd tried, questions I had and my friend Lauren to help advocate for me.

In the office I undressed and put on the starchy cotton gown. The bed I sat on was not comfortable for my back. The doctor entered and brusquely began a physical exam where he tested my strength and flexibility, and prodded me to discover which areas hurt when he pushed on them. When I lay on my stomach and he pushed on my lumbar vertebrae, I squeezed my eyes shut it hurt so badly. He proceeded to ask me questions about the meds I was taking and how the pain felt. I tried to give him the lists I had made, but when he took them he just set them aside without a glance. This same exact scenario is recounted in an auto-ethnography by Susan Greenhalgh in which she studies her experience with chronic pain and its treatment by a specialist. In her initial consultation, Greenhalgh recalls in third person:

> "She took the printed history to the appointment,
> thinking the new doctor would be keenly interested
> in her story of her medical past. But he wasn't.
> The file told the patient's history in the patient's
> own voice. The doctor wanted to start all over and
> retrieve the facts in his own format." (Greenhalgh
> 69)

In both my and Greenhalgh's experience with our specialists, our self-definition was utterly dismissed. Our stories were rendered invisible by the doctors', who promptly replaced them with their own version.

Throughout my examination, each time I tried to clarify with him a statement he had made, he interrupted me mid-sentence.

When I asked him not to interrupt me, he seemed surprised and annoyed. As the end of our session neared, I tried to cram in the questions I had written down to remember. He attempted to cut me short, saying that he had another patient waiting. I manage to say,

"My partner and I have been wanting to become pregnant. Is it possible for me to get pregnant? Will it be painful for me?"

"It could be," he said.

"Like, how painful?" I asked.

"Well, it might be excruciating," he said distractedly, as he tried to finish entering our visit description into the computer. He ordered me a C.A.T. scan and sent me on the way with the reassurance that I was "young and healthy," another statement that seemed to dismiss my pain and experience.

Later, as I returned to my car, I had a direct flashback to that night in Mexico City as I walked back to my hostel after being assaulted. I had barely been able to voice to the assualter that I was tired and wanted to go home. He proceeded to tell me how boring I was because I didn't want to party more and he was done with me. Although my internal narrative described what had taken place as a brutal violation of my mind and body, he had reduced the assault to a mere commonplace night out, albeit one with a tiresome person such as myself. In my place of vulnerability, it was easy for his language to get under my skin and for his narrative to erase and replace mine. The same was true during this visit with my physiatrist. I was vulnerable due to my pain, fear and need for medical care. This doctor was not interested in my expertise on my own body. He was dismissive of my self-identification: those things that made or took away from quality of life, my feelings, my thoughts on the cause of my pain or my beliefs about healing. Taking advantage of my vulnerability, he brushed my story aside and replaced it with his own expertise and set of values and beliefs.

In describing her anger at the overt oppression she was experiencing from and through her doctor, Greenhalgh illustrates perfectly how a person can abuse their position of power to force invisibility on another. Again in third person she writes she "was angry because she desperately needed her doctor's help, but that help was delivered in a fundamentally violent way and she had to silence her concerns about that violence to receive it" (Greenhalgh 163). In Mexico City, the building scream of my fear and anger did not burst until I was far, far away from that poisonous person. Likewise, I was not able to feel rage and to understand the way I had been fucked over by my physiatrist until some time later.

I have felt my chronic pain as a somatic translation of the times I felt oppression and the times I felt invisible. Additionally, as illustrated by my visit to the physiatrist, I have had to face new experiences of oppression and invisibility. As a person who danced since the age of three, movement was one of the primary languages I had (re)claimed to speak my presence in the world. I could use my body to create and express my identity as young, as queer, as Xicana, as female. I have felt all these identities to be denied at different times, but I at least had found a way to make them visible again to myself and to many others. However, the development of pain has left me unable to dance. Like Linda Hogan, who lost her ability to dream, I now struggle with the sensation that my "inner story" as I know it has been obliterated by this loss.

Another way I had become more visible was by finding radical community around my different identities. I often felt truly witnessed by the people I had connected with, people who also wanted to be seen in ways they had not felt growing up in our wider communities. I mostly accessed my radical community through social and physical activities like bike riding, events such as shows, dance parties and lectures, and travelling around the country. Now, my access to this community is severely limited. I am unable to ride my bike and cannot sit or stand for very long. I am often too tired from my struggle with pain during the day to attend events outside of my home. Travelling is extremely taxing to my back so I am reluctant to take trips away.

I do not know first hand the experience of oppression one has when one has a visible dis/ability. I can speak, however to the ways one is hurt, judged, denied when one has an invisible dis/ability such as chronic pain. Like going to a dance party and sitting alone on the couch even though all my friends there know I'm not CHOOSING not to dance. Like no longer being able to access bike culture and events structured around bike culture. Having people offer endless advice: I should try yoga or epsom salt baths or a million other therapies I've already tried for my pain, as though they are also experts on my body. Friends being exasperated that I have to leave a show early because my back is killing me. Or anyone at all asking how my back is but not really wanting a sincere answer. I can see their eyes begin to wander as I tell them no, it hasn't gotten better. The weight of all these experiences serves to flare my pain up more.

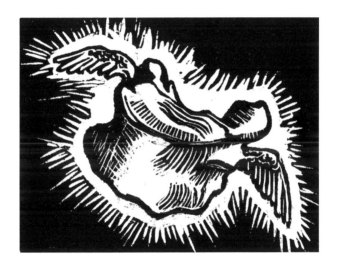

My body appears very able. I look young. I look mobile, since I can stand up and sit down and walk a block fairly easily. This breeds a lot of assumptions from people in my community. It also breeds a lot of assumptions from all the medical professionals I see every week. Many have reminded me, for no apparent reason, that I am young and healthy, just as that physiatrist did many months ago. The consequence of being treated this way is that my personal narrative, the truth I tell myself about my experience, is in constant danger of being erased by an oppressive culture. It is the perfect reflection of past traumatic events, going back generations, in which I/we have felt my/our identity invalidated to the point of seemingly not existing.

I want to say that I understand how oppression can act through good people who, through ignorance and lack of self-awareness perpetrate oppressive behaviors on those around them. I could cry for all the ways I was ableist before I had the experience myself of having a dis/ability. I think of the many times I helped organize an event without a thought to accessibility, or times I judged people for driving instead of riding a bike or not dancing at a show. I think of the girl in my dance class in college who had to have back surgery and the mere minute I took to pity her before I forgot about her entirely. Currently, these are all issues that intimately affect me. It has been a brutal education in this issue.

Like anyone suffering a loss, I have spent much of the last year in grief and anger. Each day is still a practice in coming to terms with a changing identity and the loss of old ways of speaking my truth. But I believe we will always find new ways of naming and defining ourselves and new avenues through which we can make ourselves visible in spite of and even because of pain and trauma. I have been able to find support and validation through community with other people with dis/abilities. I also finally have health care providers who I feel witness me and empower me to heal myself. I also feel that writing and making art have given me a greater voice and solidified my place in the world.

Just after viewing that painting by Frida Khalo in D.F., Mexico, I travelled to the small town of Tepoztlan to study Nahuatl, one of the more widespread languages of indigenous Mexicanos. My teacher was a very old man whom everyone called Zapata due to his remarkable likeness to the revolutionary and his wealth of wisdom. Although I learned very little of the language, I was able to do something I had longed to do for so long - feel connected to my history. Zapata and I would sit each day under a coffee tree sipping our own dark brews and he told me all about local history, herbs and healing. I befriended a little white cat who sat in my lap as we conversed. We were two people, talking, witnessing each other's stories.
On my last day in town, Zapata took me up to the ancient pyramid that towers on the mountain above Tepoztlan. From up

there, it seemed the void behind me was a little less empty and I felt my load was a bit lighter.

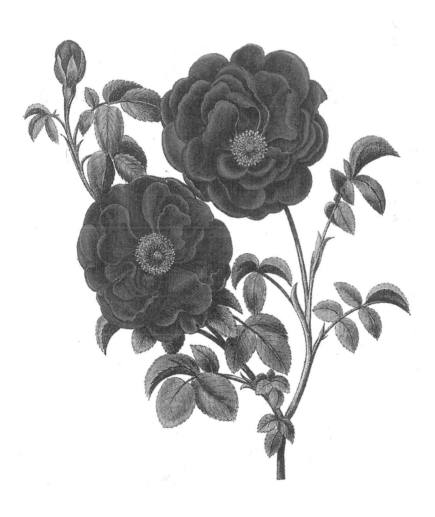

as martha graham says, the body never lies

When I was a small kid I used to get intense stomach aches frequently. They would come on like attacks and I would crumple in pain for hours. Slowly, they would dissipate. My mom was always around and I could feel her worry. Other people were around too.

We went to doctors. No medical reasons were found to be the cause. The attacks continued. When family friends visited, I might hear an aunty ask what was wrong. I would overhear my mom say to others "It's psychological." Much later in life I came to understand another word - psychosomatic.

We lived in a two-bedroom apartment in Kuwait in the mid-'80s. My mother, father, uncle, sister, and I. My parents slept in one room, and my sister and I slept on an L-shaped yellow and red bunk bed in the other bedroom. My father's brother slept on the floor in our room.

Some nights, uncle would ask me to come and sleep with him. I didn't want to, but I felt like I couldn't say no. He was an adult, an elder, a family member. All of this gave him a lot of power. I had to do what he asked me to.

When I did, he would slide his hands into my underwear. My mind always goes blank after this image.

I was 9 years old in 1990, when the Gulf War erupted and my family moved from Kuwait to India. This ended the nightmare I had been living with for two years. One night in Delhi, I was sleeping and awoke with a terrible stomach ache. I clutched my tummy and rolled around in distress, but I did not make a sound or wake anyone up. I don't know why. As I kept contorting in pain and looking at my body for the source of it, I saw reddish brown stains on the sheets. I was horrified, and rolled off the bed to the carpeted floor. Soon the blood spread to the floor, and I got scared. I was curled up in the fetal position and kept writhing different ways but couldn't make it stop. When the first light of morning started to roll in through the yellow curtains I finally alerted my mom. She explained that I had gotten my period. I didn't even know what that was, and I was stunned to learn this would happen to me for several days every month, for the next 40+ years. How come nobody had mentioned it?

I had always been a scrawny kid but within a few months I grew boobs, a belly, and a rounded butt. I received more unwanted attention, and my discomfort grew within this girl-woman body.

My first period lasted for two weeks, and then came to me like a tornado every month. I would be destroyed by excruciating pain for two to four days each time, and had to take sick days from school regularly. Doctors and nurses disbelievingly told me it was normal, and that I was too sensitive. They said that most people can go on with their regular activities after a few hours of cramps, and it shouldn't incapacitate me so. I came to dread and fear this time every month, and the onset of bleeding meant deadly pain over and over again. I kept looking for the wound, for visible signs or sources of this intensity, but there was nothing I could see or show anyone.

ʀʟʟʟʟ

In 2000, I moved to the United States as an 18-year old to study computer science at Georgia Tech. In the summer of 2002 I lived in Atlanta and I was doing an internship at Verizon Wireless. I was bored all summer, without a project or anything to do at work. I drank a lot of coffee in the break room all day long. I was 20 years old. My boss at the time was a 44-year-old White American man. He was married to a Mexican-American woman, and they had three teenage children.

One morning, I had crawled under my work desk to plug in a laptop charger. I heard a voice say "cute socks" and realized my butt and legs were sticking out from under the table. I climbed out to see my boss standing there above me, looking down, blue eyes piercing. He didn't budge. I remained frozen in my crouched position.

I started having intense stomach aches again. Frequent attacks, lasting for a few hours, slowly dissolving and leaving me drained.

On the last day of my internship, my boss asked me to go for a walk. He said, "What I have to say to you, I can't say on company grounds or I'd get fired." I knew I shouldn't go and I didn't want to, but I didn't know how to say no at that time. I had been in the U.S. for less than two years, I was a sophomore in college, and constantly felt like I stuck out as an Indian girl with an Indian accent and clothes that did not fit the American norm. This was my first off-campus work experience, and I didn't know so many things. I had been raised to obey adults, and that was often older men in power.

We went on a walk. He said, "I had a dream about you last night. We were sitting at a table across from each other. Then we kissed, with tongue." I was aghast, totally repulsed by the image, at the words coming out of his face. I didn't know what to say. I didn't say anything.

He walked me back. The internship ended. I didn't report sexual harassment. I didn't even know that that was what had happened, or that I should report it.

In my final year of college, I got politicized in a class about the high rates of sexual violence against women and girls: one out of three, one out of four. Everything was illuminated, and in that moment the course of my life was drastically altered - or perhaps it was course corrected to my true path.

After graduating with a Bachelors degree in computer science, I left the field of only 10% women and high rates of sexual harassment, and I became an anti-violence activist.

At age 26 I was divorcing a man I had loved and been with for five years. I had also discovered that I was queer. I had fallen in love with another woman. Making the decision to divorce and carrying through with it, despite immense family backlash, was one of the hardest things I have ever done.

About a year after my divorce I was home one day on my period, now an expert at pain management: heavy painkillers, a heating pad, lying down and watching TV for distraction. It was an episode of the TV series *Lost* and Sun was in labor, about to give birth. As I watched, the intensity of my own pain merged with what I was seeing on the screen. It took me a minute to realize that I wasn't just caught up in the scene. My pain was escalating rapidly. It became intolerable, and I stood up to leave for the hospital but found myself on the floor sobbing and contracted. My girlfriend drove me to the ER immediately.

That night I got my first transvaginal ultrasound, a probe inserted into my bleeding vagina to check for ovarian cysts. Apparently one had ruptured, and fluids from the cyst spilled out onto internal organs, causing inflammation and agony.

This began a period of four years where I would find myself in the ER frequently - ruptured cysts, kidney stone, even a broken rib. Along the way, I was finally diagnosed with Endometriosis, a reproductive illness that causes endometrium to grow outside the uterus where it proliferates with the hormonal cycle, has no way to be shed, dies internally and becomes scar tissue, binding internal organs together and causing acute and chronic pain over time. Endometriosis occurs in about 10% of the female-bodied population, but the average delay in diagnosis is approximately ten years. It was fifteen years for me, despite all the textbook signs - early onset of menstruation, irregular cycles, extreme pain, dysmenorrhea (extreme PMS). I believe this delay in diagnosis is a result of sexism in the medical industry that severely minimizes the pain that women and girls express, especially when it's invisible.

There is no certain cause of Endometriosis, and no certain cure. There are only theories of origin and treatments to manage symptoms. One of the origin theories is that Endometriosis is a manifestation of sexual trauma, and another theory is that it is passed on from mother to child in utero, and can pass on the mother's sexual or reproductive trauma as well.

From the wholeness of my life experiences, I have come to believe the following things:

- Sexual violence is an often-invisible trauma, and I believe that, for me, developing Endometriosis is connected to surviving sexual violence.
- Chronic pain is invisible yet can be debilitating in extremely visible ways. Endometriosis allowed my body to manifest the pain I had often silenced.
- Illness and pain have taught me great patience, deepened my spirituality, and also compelled me to live life in a more balanced way. It taught me to listen to my body's truth, and to follow its wisdom.
- Chronic illness, pain, and disability taught me the greatest of life lessons - to ask for and receive support. My relationships are truer and stronger as a result, and I am so grateful to all the people who taught me this. It was not easy.

The long journey of healing has led me to develop the following beliefs about health and wellness:

- Physical, mental, emotional, spiritual, environmental, and community health are connected.
- There are seven core elements to holistic well-being:
  - REST - adequate and nourishing sleep and downtime.
  - NUTRITION - balanced & seasonally grounded intake of nutrients.
  - WATER - full hydration for cleansing and cell rejuvenation.
  - MOVEMENT - physical movement of all realms and speeds, to strengthen, generate energy and excitement, and also for mental health and happiness.
  - BREATH - Deep breathing for self-containment and fullness, meditation, calming and relaxing, and increased mindfulness.
  - LAUGHTER - Fun, joy, laughter and lightness to lift our spirits and heal our bodies and souls.
  - CONNECTION - We are happier in genuine caring connection with other human beings.
- Having a positive approach changes everything - i.e. believing the best about people and situations, putting energy into building people up.

- Love is healing, and two very significant forms are time/attention and physical touch/affection.
- Faith plays a powerful role in healing, in the journey and the outcomes.
- Trauma can be stored in us from things that happened to us, to our family of origin or the family we were raised in, and also from our ancestral and collective experiences. This aspect of healing takes a lot of energy, time, and support and guidance, and firm intention and commitment. Doing this work serves our future ancestors.
- Doing something we love everyday keeps us connected to our joy and our center, which is a powerful compass for well-being.
- Everything happens for a reason, and everything happens for the best in its whole interconnectedness. We can't always see or know that, but trusting that allows us to lean into the positives of the current moment, discern how to make the best of it, learn meaningful lessons and move forward.

For me, pain has been a teacher guiding me towards my path. It has also given me the motivation to heal from emotional trauma, and strengthen my body through physical therapy. This doesn't mean there aren't days with extreme pain, or lack of mobility, but my spirits are joyful, I have incredible community, clarity of life purpose, and I have seen my strength. I wish the same for all who live with pain. ♥

seasoning

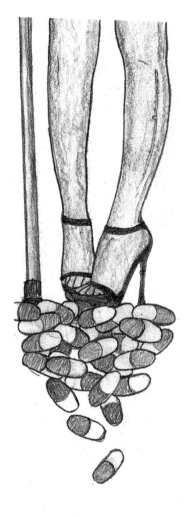

That was the winter I stopped wearing bras (again); bought sheer black nylons for the first time since childhood churchood - two at a time because my leg hair turned friction into runs. Two at a time on sale because I knew one pair would be the ones with all of the widening roads up my thighs and sometimes I didn't care about runs, others I did.

That was the spring I started looking for my femme uniform; started to build my identity as a "femme crip of colour." I'd spent the last year of my illness in a miserable state and wanted to strut out of my house, cane in one hand and anxiety meds - in a fabulous bag, in the other.

It was the year I stopped leaving the house, but when I did it was never without earrings and lipstick. When I switched what jewelry I could from silver to gold because that's what my mother wore.

The spring I went to California and fell in love with the me I became there. I wore dresses, tights, smiles and warm skin for ten days, only to come home to a hail storm and my own tears.

That was the autumn, the winter, the spring I fucked everyone but my partner because my cock-trauma had made a surprise visit and I could barely imagine a bulge without trembling. I had sex in ways that disregarded the state of my bones, muscles, nerves - make-believing that I could do all the twists and turns and jumps of energetic loving. I pretended I was my 20 year old self with stamina for days and muscles like putty. While I tried to screw my memories back where they came from, my body screamed and pleaded with me to stop. Aching and sore, wincing at the slightest movement, I ended my coital carnival just in time for the subsequent cerebral unraveling (otherwise knows as nervous breakdown).

The spring the psychiatrist said my "multiple problems" could be helped by more pills, but the flaws in my personality were up to me. "Good luck, Ms. Gayle," he'd said without lifting his head to look at me. When I saw that doctor again, I remember coming in the door and him asking, "How are you?" Still getting settled in my seat, putting my bags and bike helmet on the floor, I'd said: "I'm fine." To that he responded, sternly and with irritation in his voice "That is how you respond to other people. When I ask you how you're doing - you tell me the truth."

That spring I asked repeatedly, to be referred to a rheumatologist to rule out/in certain conditions. Each time I was deferred to conversations about my mental "health." In short: the doctor thought I was making all the pain up.

I wrote him this letter:

Dear Dr. D:

A year ago I came to you suffering from withdrawal symptoms as a result of an accidental abrupt cessation of the medication Cymbalta which you had prescribe to me three months prior. I explained that after my time on the drug, I was not pleased with its effects on my body and asked to be removed. Instead of listening to my request you suggested I increase my dose. At the time I was extremely ill and vulnerable. I had to be accompanied to your office because I could barely stand or walk from the pain and vertigo I was experiencing. Perhaps had I been feeling better I would have further protested, but, as you had been my doctor for almost 10 years at that point - I trusted you and left with the script in hand.

At no time in your initial prescribing of this drug or subsequent increase did you spend any time informing me of the severe side effects of both being on the drug and coming off of it. You also failed to mention the high cost.

Since that visit my physical and mental health have deteriorated drastically and I believe some of that can be attributed to this medication.

Some of the symptoms that have appeared or reappeared are: major depression, anxiety, insomnia, low sex drive, suicidal thoughts, self harming, dissociative episodes including altered personalities, dizziness, nausea, headaches and mood swings.

In combination with the decline of my health these symptoms contributed to my need to leave my full time job, thus losing the benefits that provided me with the ability to afford the meds in the first place.

Since I have been disabled by chronic pain and mental illness I have begun to live in poverty and on social assistance. My unpredictable mental heath makes it difficult to seek full time work and working part time does not allow for much income in this expensive city.

This medication is expensive, dangerous, and, above all, not working. I have sought numerous avenues in an effort to get off of it and all have pointed back to the prescribing physician - you.

I am going to ask again, demand for your assistance in withdrawing from this medication. If you cannot provide that help, please direct me to someone who can.

I have been really disappointed with your level of care and will consider seeking an alternate physician in the future.

Thank You,
Melannie

The spring and spring and spring that seem to lay pregnant with summer forever; teasing me as I waited for the sweat-dripping season I believed would push me out of my madness into a normalcy I could only anticipate but not remember.

Now, as humidity moistens my brown skin and the sun darkens me like bread in an oven, I continue to wait for the ebb and flow of my wild mind to slow down. To stop crashing waves into the shore, so I can have a respite.

I still have not seen a rheumatologist; I have yet to find a doctor who hasn't told me I am making it up. Even if I never get an answer as to why I strain to breathe deeply, why seemingly unknown movements create ripples of stabbing pain throughout my body, why walking for more than two blocks causes my body to seize and my brain to thud in an effort to keep going: This is the body I have.

She has been hurt, scarred, and manipulated in her time, but also squeezed, hugged, tickled, kissed and loved softly. And I will hold onto those quiet, kind moments with everything I have, red fingernails and all, for as long as I can.

even as the small me

I remember where I was sitting when I had one of those moments of clarity where the circumstances and the elements lurking as corners and backdrops of the mind suddenly ripen to a point of connection. I was sitting on a rock. A particular rock in a pile of rocks, which form a sea defence, near my mum's house - not the rock I habitually sat on, but one further back. It was summer or early autumn. I think I had began recording a song I was writing, but finally ended up just talking to some kind of machine - my tablet, or dictaphone. I have searched for the recording but it's disappeared into an electronic nowhere.

I remember feeling validated by the machine's silent acceptance of my words. I could say what I couldn't say to any human, I could talk freely, without formulating my stream of consciousness to please or entertain or not offend its specific self. And I could say things I couldn't say to myself, I could go somehow further than I could in the confined space of my interior thought process. I don't remember the precise order of thoughts evolving or what triggered what, but it occurred to me that my chronic pain was precisely preventing me from doing that which I most wanted to do, which was play music. However, before I developed the pain, I already had big barriers to fulfilling my desire for creative expression, in the form of a lack of confidence, a complex form of shame that attacked me if ever I performed. I wrote songs in secret and while I internally believed in my work, I was paralysed when it came to taking it into the world. This was a source of great frustration and drained my energy as every blockage does. I sat thinking about how unfortunate it was that I now had not only one really significant barrier, but two. This created a situation in which if I was having a good day mood-wise, feeling confident and energetic and not ashamed, and the opportunity arose to play music the chances that I would be in a physical state to do so were slim. Likewise I might be physically capable one day but in the grips of my shame complex. However, because I knew that I had psychosocial reasons to turn down a jam or whatever, if someone asked me to play music and I felt resistance in myself, I often pushed myself out of habit, even if I knew my body was not in a strong way - I

wanted to avoid the self flagellation that would follow should
I not participate, which, even when the reason was physical,
automatically blamed my psychology if I didn't participate in
something I wanted to. And that exacerbated my chronic pain, in
a vicious cycle.

The reasons for not doing the thing I love became all mixed
up, complicating any possible route through. Before the pain,
I was working on my confidence, and in a process of learning
self-acceptance. And before my pain went into its worst phase,
I had a very good phase in which I finished making a harp, and
began teaching myself how to play it. I remember taking it to
the beach, singing to it, hugging it between my legs and arms. I
loved it, it gave me an ownership of sound I had never felt before
and I knew with this instrument I could build a sound I felt was
mine. With the onset of severe pain, everything collapsed in a
slagheap. Increasingly I couldn't do basic tasks or look after
myself, let alone the things I enjoyed. I lost my job, the roof over
my head, and learnt more about the depths of intimacy to which
fierce individualism reaches, and the way it disguises itself in the
eyes of the independent.

As I sat and ruminated on how my physical pain and shame
got mixed together in relation to performing, I discovered the
possibility that my physical disability was actually caused
by my psychosocial disability, along many indirect routes, all
converging together in the pain. I realised that I could have been
disabled in any number of ways, but this specific pain impacted
music especially. I also had vocal problems associated with neck
tension and pain. I realised that after my accidents, I could have
healed well but instead I developed chronic myofascial pain, and
why?

Was it because of my posture; my collapsed posture, due to my
low energy, due to my on and off depression? My collapse cut
off circulation to my arm, and made my breathing shallow, thus
starving the damaged tissues of the oxygen and nutrients they
needed to heal. Because of my damaged immune response, also
related to my mental health struggles? The immune system is
deeply implicated in healing after injury. Because of the way I
attacked the piano when I played, the way my upper body filled
with tension when I played the guitar, because of how I strained
to create the right sound, out of a lack of confidence in my
abilities? Because of the way I didn't trust my own body when it
was hurting and go home from a bike tour, but instead continued,

believing that going home would be giving in to a psychological complex? How I consistently pushed through pain and could not get the hang of pacing myself to give my injury time to heal, out of fear that my good mood would not last, and that if I stopped working on my project now I would not come back to it? Because of my rebellious and passionate spirit that refused to impose moderation on itself whilst in the grip of inspiration? Because of my internalisation of clichés about suffering for art; because of the way I had stayed alive through extremely painful times through my art, and thus saw it as the most important secret thing I would never concede, more important than my health, the insistent voice of my body?

If I hadn't been a person so erratic in my moods, so prone to momentary elations followed by fatigue and bad moods, I wouldn't have felt the need to grasp joy so tightly when it appeared. I saw how the mechanics of my whole self had led to this situation, and how I would have to change my whole self if there was to be any hope to move out of it. I saw how my physical disability was in fact a precipitation of some kind of energetic contradiction that I had already been the owner of. Not, of course, the only logical outcome, but a logical outcome of the mass of things that was my life history.

Simple pain tells us simply what to do, like get our hands out of the fire, or not walk while our leg is broken. Devyn Starlanyl writes in her book *Fibromyalgia and Chronic Myofascial Pain: A Survival Manual*, that non-chronic pain is life preserving while chronic pain is life destroying. I can definitely relate to the feeling of being drained of life by pain. But I think chronic pain can be read as life preserving too, as our bodies telling us what we need to do. However as it is more complex it has to be decoded and sometimes its messages are counterintuitive.

When we want to explain complex concepts to each other, we use metaphors, similes and comparisons to evoke the meaning that we are trying to communicate. In a similar way, might chronic pain be the way we experience the body using its own basic mechanisms to talk to us - even when its message is more complex? Might that be what is happening when we have pain that seems to be illogical, that won't go away? And when viewed like this, as a coded communication from our bodies, the unconscious, or something outside of us, is it possible to decode our chronic pain?

Also, who is talking to us through the language of our pain? If our pain is a coded message from our bodies to our minds, from our unconscious, or the collective unconscious, to ourselves, it is impossible to view it as our enemy. But at the same time, if I have understood correctly that my pain has developed partially in response to my shame, a shame imposed on me by interpersonal and societal violence; do I have to befriend shame too? That is hard.

pain as oppressor

Shame is an oppressor; I cannot see it otherwise. For me the word shame denotes a kind of fear of social punishment, fear of the consequences of social ostracization; one of the most powerful tools of oppressive systems. My shame was internalized through a combination of bullying and gendered violence that I experienced, in addition to familial shame I inherited. I can think of my chronic pain as the result of my various diverging responses to that shame, finally colliding and becoming a single entity - in the same way that literal myofascial trigger points form. This makes it essentially an internal representation of the societal poison of shame, leading me to understand the pain itself as an oppressive force too; an externally imposed, foreign thing within me that I need to overcome or expel.

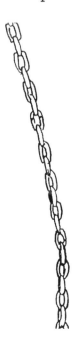

WHAT IT FEELS LIKE *it has the feeling of a kind of anchor, a blunt metal anchor that has materialised inside my flesh, heavy and cutting and dull at the same time and dragging me down, while the people skip around the surface in their little motorboats, unseeing, and some glide by in kayaks and canoes, who see me and look at me with sympathy but cannot pull me in because they would risk upturning their delicately balanced vessels, and i can see how if they worked together they could help me, if they attracted the attention of the larger boats and somehow got them to help me, but they don't, and i'd rather if they didn't see me at all, because now i am ashamed to be looked at with those eyes as i am dragged down, i don't want those*

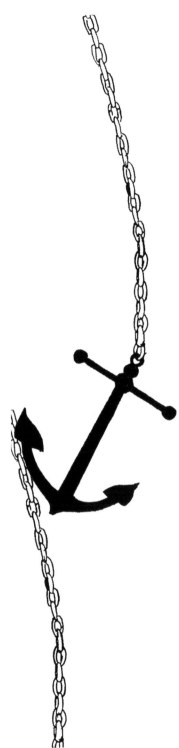

people to feel they have any power over me, i know how even the well meaning abuse power, because i mean well. so now i have stopped trying not to drown, i am willing, i want to be taken right to the depths where i am safe from those boats chopping around and those pitying people, i want either to be alone or surrounded only by people who have known the same sorrow and who won't harass and incite shame in me with their expectations, their lack of understanding, their wavering between sympathy and judgment, their pity, their rejection.

and so now how can i see the pain as my oppressor, that anchor which has dragged me down, which now holds me here at the bottom of the ocean where there is a kind of peace, although i can't breathe? had someone dragged me up into their boat i would have said, 'look, here is this thing which is inside me but it is not me, it is hurting me, please help me get it out, the edges have grafted with my nasty scarred up muscle but still i think it can be gotten out'. now i have gotten to the bottom of the sea, it is hard to imagine what would happen if i were able to separate myself from this thing, though how i would do that down here in the water without help god only knows; would my body, de-weighted under this water just collapse, would it float up to the surface, weak and light averse, to just drift around in the tide? i can't cut it out even if i wanted to, and yet I don't want to accept that i am living in a deep isolation eternally married to an oppressive complex.

Can the pain be something other than oppressor?

Pain as healer, pain as teacher, pain as god

If pain is a teacher, where do we go and what do we do when we are incapable of learning, of integrating its lessons? We stay where we are, or we run away; either way, we continue to suffer. That is why so many of us suffer. There are many ways we can be incapable of changing our lives to integrate lessons in this world. Our capability or lack thereof here relates intrinsically to our disempowerment at the hands of the current global socioeconomic system. I see it as a fact that the more privilege we are able to leverage, the easier it generally will be to integrate necessary changes.

For me, my chronic illness hit at what seemed like the worst possible time: right after I had left university, and was working out where to go and what to do. I didn't have the structure of university life, which provided purpose, activity, and community (if to an inadequate extent for my needs). And I hadn't yet worked out where I was going to get those things from. Had I had a clear path or structure in my life to hold together or adapt to my new needs, things would have been infinitely more straightforward. Illness doesn't choose the best time to strike for our own growth. It strikes when it can take our split selves no longer. When we have worn it down to its last nerve, I suppose.

If the forces of life, the universe and everything are what whacks us, pain is no more the whack itself than it is our body's response to that whack. And our body's response to that whack is our body telling us to move or somehow change.

A part of me has come to view pain as the place where conflicting forces meet. The forces that animate the universe meet themselves in another form; a conscious form that has been intricately twisted and refined through millennia of evolution. Pain is the feeling of that ongoing manipulation; it is the feeling of a change being violently forced upon us. This change is what we are; it is how we exist as conscious beings.

> *"When an apprentice gets hurt, or complains of being tired, the workmen and peasants have this fine expression: "It is the trade entering his body." Each time that we have some pain to go through, we can say to ourselves quite truly that it is the universe, the order and*

*beauty of the world, and the obedience of God that are
entering our body"* - Simone Weil

At times I feel that the forces that are hurting me and spurring
me to change are in fact crushing me, that my body and spirit
will not evolve but will instead be lost under the wave; that I am
inadequate as a human, and an animal, as a conscious creature
to the task of survival. Sometimes I am able to console myself
by connecting with a larger truth; that life is only a competition
from the standpoint of the individual. I imagine that all the
alternative beings that could have existed in my place in this
world, the children my parents could have had, their small
spirits are all part of my spirit; maybe as we grow older, we
grow more conscious because all the conscious beings that die at
every stage get added to us like drops of water joining a stream.
The people I know who have died young, my childhood pets; my
grandma; the creatures that die are not gone and have not failed
at anything. So I can see that this pain is very powerful and not
be scared. And sometimes I feel like I have grown, I will not be
destroyed, even as an individual person, even as the small me. I
suppose all of these things are true.

What is amazing is that we can sometimes even glimpse the way
that our pain is forcing us to grow, as it happens; we can glimpse
how our lives were not in harmony with those larger forces.

> *"I have heard it said that illness is an attempt to escape
> the truth. I suspect it is actually an attempt to embody the
> whole truth, to remember all of ourselves."*

Which part of myself have I somehow left behind, blocked out or
forgotten? In her beautiful book, *The Alchemy of Illness*, Kat Duff
relates to the reader her experience of chronic fatigue immune
dysfunction syndrome, and how she was able to draw meaning
from its depths. I was struck by her account of a dream in which
she realises that her exhaustion is a mechanism preventing her
from becoming completely dissociated from herself:

> *"I had a dream the night before I received my CFIDS
> diagnosis and learned there was no cure for it; the dream
> showed me how my incest recovery would continue
> through the agency of my illness. In that dream I belonged
> to a group of women incest survivors who met weekly
> to blaze trails through rough wooded territory. We hung
> little mirrors from the branches of trees to see better and
> tried very hard to do it right; even so, we kept getting lost,*

confused, and separated, and ended up fighting amongst ourselves. Finally, we stopped and asked ourselves: How can we keep from losing it like this, from dissociating and splitting apart? As soon as we asked the question, a wise woman appeared and demonstrated a simple spiritual exercise for pulling ourselves back together and cultivating the self possession of the masters; to collapse with exhaustion. We proceeded to do exactly that, each one of us dropping to the floor with a loud sigh, then, one by one, we told the stories of our lives, our deepest hurts, regrets and yearnings. As we connected with ourselves and each other, a deep calm enveloped and united us."

Because we rarely hear accounts from ill people of their illness, because the reality of illness is that it disorders the very parts of us that would otherwise be engaged in remembering, explaining, and categorising it, *"illness remains a wilderness.... it may play an important, even necessary, role in the ecology of the whole."*

Societally, we are living in times that seek to fragment us, disengaging our energies from our capacity to calibrate and direct ourselves. Duff's suggestion that the agency of an illness itself could be what does the healing - that what we experience as the illness itself is not only what can teach us how to heal, but may be the actual healing happening - feels important. I think integrating this understanding can reconnect us to a broader sense of meaning.

As in homeopathy, a particular illness may warrant a solution that balances not only that illness or manifestation of illness in a person, but also the symptoms and tendencies they are not attempting to address, and may not even have recognised. In a larger sense, our illnesses can be viewed as the beginning of a self healing process that nature is living; our attempts to heal in a way that integrates the lessons of illness may continue this work of nature, which is correcting itself in ways and on levels that we do not have access to.

For me on a personal level, the best solution I have found for my pain has been meditation, connecting with spirituality, and bodywork. My pain simultaneously forced me to inhabit my body and the present moment, as one cannot avoid when one is in pain, and intensified my desire to escape it. Escaping the frightening vulnerability of my body is what I had been doing for years - as pain has dragged me back into it, I have had to acknowledge that leaving my body behind only leaves it, and thus myself, more vulnerable to damage. So I have to learn a new way of living, in my body. This doesn't make pain go away, but it prevents me from creating more pain by doing things that exacerbate it while dissociating. And at the same time, it brings me back to the truth of myself, from where I can act authentically and do what I mean to in the world; contribute and not blindly hurt other people and living things. I hope that it will bring me more and more fully into peace with myself and the world. I have known this flow and peace and I want to live there. But there is a lot to integrate. In order to make this kind of integration possible, we all need to plunge into the work of undoing our individualism and isolation and building true communities of healing.

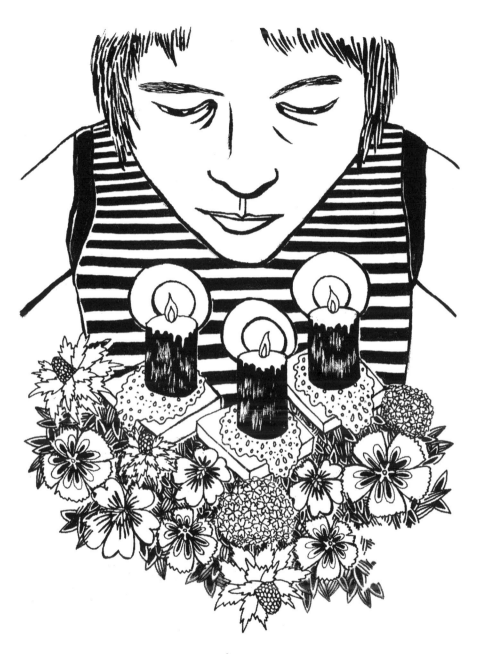

on self care

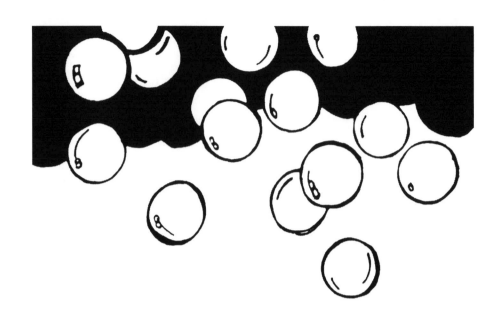

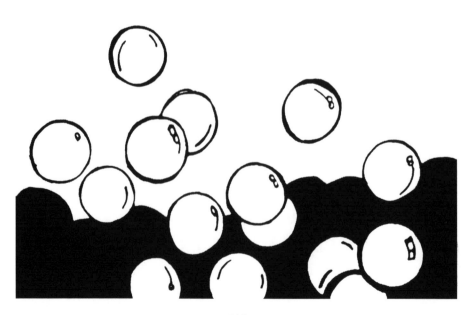

Karen Hixon

beyond the bubble bath
a harm reduction guide to self care

I first heard the phrase "self care" while working as a sexual assault advocate in 1998. It was my first professional job, and I had absolutely no idea what I was getting into. While we often mentioned self care at my agency, it was rare to see solid modeling of it. What did self care really look like? I knew it had to be more than just a bubble bath at the end of the day. And I was often confused that it was my total responsibility to implement self care practices, when, in fact, the policies and work culture seemed to be setting me up for burnout regardless of my individual decisions. Fourteen months after starting, I was suffering from some significant symptoms of trauma exposure. I've been thinking about, reading about and discussing the concept and practice of self care since that first experience with burnout.

Many people warn we can't take care of others if we don't take care of ourselves. In some ways, this is totally accurate because we will eventually reach a crisis point or stray far from our intended goals for helping others. However, many people manage to take care of others without taking good care of themselves. Sometimes the impacts are obvious and other times quite hidden to outside observers. The reality is that it can be hard to take care of ourselves. We'd rather spend the energy on other people. Many things get in the way of taking care of ourselves and being able to care for others. We don't have the time. We don't have the resources. We feel selfish. We are overwhelmed at how to begin. Adding to the complexity is the sense that at times, people in our community need care regardless of our ability to give.

In modern society, there exists a baseline amount of anxiety and stress and a lingering sense of being overwhelmed. Work, school, errands, chores and simple maintenance of life take a certain level of energy and time. Add to that the additional demands of children, creative projects, single parenting, second jobs, care of other ill family members and a desire to care for our communities, the animals and the environment ... talk about overwhelming! If you also have an experience of chronic pain, chronic illness, are living with a disability or have mental health difficulties as part of your experience, then self care becomes an additional necessity (and challenge) rather than a "when-I-have-time-for-it" luxury.

Further complicating our relationship to self care is that we can judge ourselves very harshly for not tending to our own needs. When we aren't feeling so well others often ask us if we are taking care of ourselves. There can be some veiled judgment (or perhaps our own projections) that we are to blame for our current state because we didn't do it right. Our own ebbs and flows of emotional struggle or physical pain can also make it difficult to engage with and maintain self care. The heartache of tending to yourself when you feel broken, unfixable and in pain is challenging. A flare up can really challenge your commitment to yourself.

It helps me to view self-care as somewhat aspirational - I know the ideal way I'd take care of myself, my family and my community if I had endless time and abundant resources to do so. I often say that I could make it my full time job (and perhaps it should be)! Over the years, I've learned that my constitution along with the kind of work I do require that I take care of myself. If I'm not intentional about the amount of time I devote to self care, my body will hurt, anxiety will flare up and I will become resentful of the very activities I choose to spend my time on. I will be crabby with those I love the most. I will start complaining endlessly. I'm not so fun when I don't take care of myself. If I don't take the time to do essential chores that create calmness in my space, schedule important appointments or hang outs and ensure my schedule is reasonable, it becomes overwhelming to balance everything.

My reflections on the topic of self care along with my observations of my own patterns have led me to utilize harm reduction theory as a basis for formulating a self care plan. *Meeting myself where I am* (the essential core of harm reduction theory) seems a more reasonable way to contextualize self care. I know I'm not going to be able to take care of myself perfectly all the time and I will fall off the self care wagon. So why not give myself some room to do the best I can at any given time instead of trying to live up to some rigid expectation of taking perfect care of myself? Perhaps this will allow us more room to support others as well.

As I hear more and more people in my community talk of being extremely busy and overextended, I hope we will all take the time out to consider what actually works best for us. What kinds of activities make us feel the most restored, inspired and creative? What kind of schedule allows us to be present for both others and ourselves? What kind of nurturing do we truly need to be able to do the kind of work we want to do? How do we create awareness in our communities regarding the need to tend to each other? What follows are some possible suggestions on utilizing a harm reduction framework to activate your self care. I've also included three visual examples of self care plans. Please take what is useful to you and leave the rest behind. I'm keenly aware of the inherent paradox of focusing on self care. Others have suggested we move away from self care to communities of care. I agree. And let's start where we are and build an increasing level of awareness and skill regarding giving and receiving care. The challenge to move away from self care is best put by Yashna Maya Padamsee "Self-care, as it is framed now, leaves us in danger of being isolated in our struggle and our healing. Isolation of yet another person, another injustice, is a notch in the belt of Oppression. A liberatory care practice is one in which we move beyond self-care into caring for each other."

ACTIVATING & MAINTAINING SELF CARE

1. You will not be consistent. Don't stress it!

Our best-laid plans are always interrupted. We have a bad day (or week). We go on vacation. Friends come into town. Our family visits. We have too much work to do and taking care of ourselves seems like more work. We have a flare up and we have to put our plan on hold. Don't let this stop you from re-starting whenever the time feels right. Let go of how you didn't go to the gym for two weeks or you avoided doing your exercises while your friends were visiting. Let go of the idea that your plan will someday be perfectly adhered to, no matter what.

2. Start today/Do One Thing.

Don't think of *all* the things you'd like to care for yourself, just focus on one thing. Meet yourself where you are. Yes, you might not be living up to your ideal plans, but you can start making better choices at any point. Ate a bad breakfast? What choices can you make about your lunch? Skipped physical therapy this week? Set up your next appointment. Don't let one decision or one bad day sabotage you from doing the next best thing for yourself.

3. Punishment doesn't work.

You cannot control, dominate or judge yourself into good self care. We are human and we rebel when control is the dominant paradigm. It's more common for us to beat ourselves up for what we are not doing rather than celebrate the small victories. Try to drum up some compassion or kindness for yourself as the basis for taking care of yourself. Watch that nasty voice in your head that tells you, "I should be...." "I can't believe I didn't..." "Wow, another day without....." Be mindful of the running narrative. Flip the script. Be gentle.

4. Plant flowers instead of pulling weeds.

I find it much easier to add good stuff rather than working to remove all the not so good stuff I'm doing. I might not be willing to eliminate bad television from my life but I can add a walk after dinner. Too much coffee? Add some water to the regimen. Put your focus on something you want to expand. Slowly, the flowers take over!

5. Self care is multi-faceted, complex and even paradoxical.

At times it means not going to yoga because you'd be more nourished by hanging out with a friend. It can mean that you need alone time, social time or medical care. At times, you might need time to self-reflect, at others, to be distracted. Be flexible with yourself and embrace the irony that anti-self care is self care sometimes.

6. Have a plan.

It is very difficult to take care of yourself if you don't know what you need. Everyone is different, and I find that I need different things at different times in my life. I try to check in with myself often because my needs change, sometimes on a daily basis. I wake up feeling like I need to go to acupuncture, but later, I find joy and wellness in sitting at the coffee shop writing letters to friends. Take some time to make a plan and occasionally put a self care plan review on your agenda.

7. Consider how to support your self-care plan.
Consider whom in your family or circle of friends you would like to have support your self care plan. What, if any, specific prompts, questions or words of encouragement would you appreciate from loved ones? How can you remind yourself (without guilt) that your self-care plan is available and ready? Is it something you'd like to tell people about? Hang up in your room? Would this be helpful to discuss with a professional counselor, social worker or other healer?

8. Ask for Help/Ask to Help.
We are very fearful of burdening others to the point that we suffer in isolation. It is very difficult to ask for help and that difficulty increases if you are in a vulnerable place. In my experience, when I do ask for help from trusted friends and family, I'm often met with kindness and generosity. I want to live in community where I can ask for what I need without guilt and shame and trust that people will be honest about their ability to support me. I want to create those communities of care. I want someone to bring me a casserole when I am having a hard time. I want to do those things for others, too.

BRAINSTORMING CATEGORIES FOR YOUR SELF CARE PLAN:

- ☐ Chores/Errands
- ☐ To Do Lists/Goal Setting
- ☐ Sleep/Rest/Relaxation
- ☐ Exercise/Movement
- ☐ Activities that support your work/Career
- ☐ Journaling
- ☐ Creativity/Art/Crafts/Writing

- ☐ Hobbies
- ☐ Spiritual/Religious Practices
- ☐ Alone time
- ☐ Adventures
- ☐ Vacations
- ☐ Supportive people/Hang Outs with Loved Ones
- ☐ Attitudes/Philosophies/Words/Quotes/Intentions
- ☐ Dates/Sex
- ☐ Food/Meal Planning
- ☐ Supplements/Medication
- ☐ Healing/Medical Appointments
- ☐ Communication with Loved Ones
- ☐ Financial Needs/Goals

EXAMPLES OF SELF CARE PLANS:

These are just a starting place! Get creative! Make your plans as simple or elaborate as you want. Include others in the creation of your plan. Copy it for those in your support system. Make it work for you.

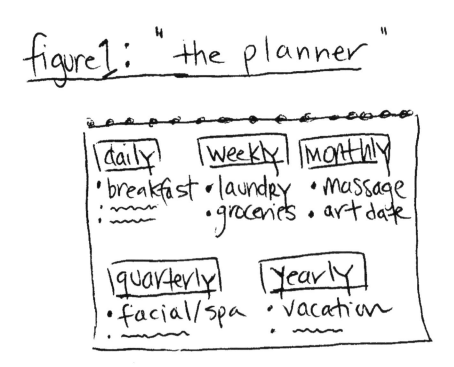

figure 1: "the planner"

daily
- breakfast

weekly
- laundry
- groceries

monthly
- massage
- art date

quarterly
- facial/spa

yearly
- vacation

figure 2: "the collage"

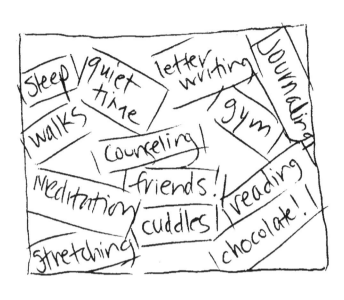

Sleep | quiet time | letter writing | Journaling
walks | gym
Counseling
Meditation | friends! | reading
cuddles | chocolate!
Stretching

figure 3: "ideal pie"

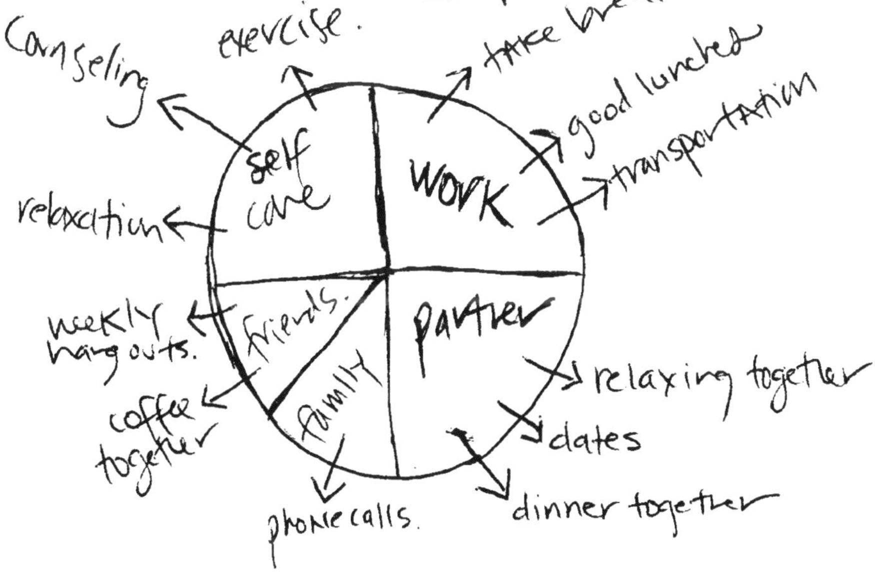

Counseling
exercise.
take breaks
good lunches
transportation

self care
WORK

relaxation

weekly hang outs.
friends.
partner

coffee together
family
relaxing together
dates
dinner together

phone calls.

Jonah Aline Daniel

paper in your hands

"everything is like paper in my hands,"
you marvel cautiously at the lightness and ease
with which your changing body lifts and carries
climbs, grips, holds, hits
everything seems so delicate
its so effortless to push and pull
restrain
restrict
crumble
crumple
without effort
the weight of the world
like paper in your hands

i move from lying down to a standing up position in
   physical therapy
and fatigue washes through my body
pools
stays
exhausted by the simple act of holding myself upright

the weight of my own limbs
the relentless pulling tension
from the origin of the winding impeded roads that enervate
   my arms
all the way through to the tips of my fingers
my body speaks to me about the labor of being awake

i cringe at the pain of holding my pen, my fork
dispensing my own medicine
of holding up my own head
i wonder where our common ground is
and what there is to learn

...

testosterone crashed through your veins
each wednesday morning
and you crashed through the world
crashed through my life
with your relentlessly positive outlook
your unwavering, glowing witness
your logical explanations and solutions

but there was no room for grief
for fear
for doubt
for defeat
the world a procession of practical next steps
you needing so desperately to fix something
fix someone
i needing a fix

but there is nothing wrong with me
nothing that needs fixing
my pain is a part of me
my opportunity to be self responsive
to gather information about my boundaries and my needs
to learn the excruciating lessons of what it means to live
  in a body

i tell my friends my shocking realizations this winter
"this is the only body that I have!" i say.
"i am the only one that has this body!"
there is no fix, no escape
the work is mine
the work of accepting the body that I have
and learning to live
learning to love

who can meet me here?
just as i am

holding a delicate balance between acceptance and resignation
between a calm presence with what I have and a trust that
  I can heal
that I can transform
riding the highs of my victories and the crushing defeat of loss

and limitation
whole and hurting
shedding skin
open hearted
submerged in my depths
steeped in the intimacy of being my own caregiver
who can meet me here?
able to care for me and receive my care
just as we are

saying yes

I almost didn't go to the river today. Despite record high temperatures sending all of my friends to cool off in nearby bodies of water, my first impulse when asked along was to stay behind. Invite me somewhere and nine times out of ten the phrase *I can't do that* runs across my mind. Years of living with chronic pain have cultivated a pretty strict inner dialog. I cautiously dismantle the possible physical situation I could be put in for each proposed event - *How long would I be in the car? That sounds like a lot of sitting. What is the trail to the beach like? Walking on uneven surfaces is hard on my back...* - I say no because I am afraid that saying yes will increase my pain.

Talking myself out of participation has become like second nature to me, but when I take a step back I am saddened by all that I have given up to avoid experiencing pain. In trying to take another look at this I have gained some helpful tools from the workbook *Living Beyond Your Pain: Using Acceptance and Commitment Therapy to Ease Chronic Pain* by Joanne Dahl and Tobias Lundgren.

The book builds itself on the idea that, for people living with chronic pain, seeking pain reduction can be a trap. Most of us have spent years looking for a solution to our pain, the magic combination of medications or therapies that will alleviate our suffering, and that solution has eluded us. The energy we put into this search, the feelings of failure and disappointment of never finding relief, the psychological difficulty of the fight, the book argues, perpetuate our suffering.

Using a combination of written and mindfulness based exercises drawn from Acceptance and Commitment Therapy, this book challenges its readers to discover what they value and move toward a life more aligned to those values. Rather than trying to avoid or control pain, a force that is ultimately and frustratingly uncontrollable for most of us, *Living Beyond You Pain* suggests that, with committed action, it is possible to live life more fully than our pain might be telling us we can.

One helpful piece of the book for me is a distinction that the authors make between two kinds of pain, what they call "clean" and "dirty" pain. Clean pain is purely physical, the sensations our body uses to tell us something is wrong. Dirty pain is physical pain polluted with ideas. It is the mud we get stuck in trying to fix things. It is the way that our minds react to the pain we are experiencing, the judgments and adjustments we make to accommodate that pain.

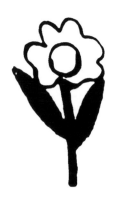

For me, pain comes as the result of an injury to my back. Still daily but not as acute as it once was, my physical pain ranges from modest dull ache to full nerve flare. Sometimes manifesting as muscle stiffness, weakness, or cramps, other times vulnerable but released, loose, and flexible. Over time, as my physical pain persisted without successful medical intervention, loss came with it and 'muddied' it up: loss of opportunities, of the ability to support myself, loss of a sense of self, of confidence in my ability to heal, loss of important friendships, of connection to community... and the exhaustion that comes from reacting to, and fighting against injury set in a major way.

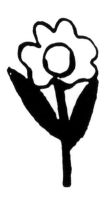

My head is full, and still runs wild amassing rules as I experience pain - *I should not sit for long periods of time, I should not bend, lift, and twist. I should not do super bouncy physical stuff like running or riding a bike. If I am going to be doing a lot of standing or walking I need supportive and sensible shoes. I'm better off if I change positions frequently, and I need to take breaks to lay down a lot* - these rules about body mechanics enter my mind when I make everyday decisions. I follow them as a means of control, even when I know that breaking them doesn't necessarily produce or increase my pain. I tell myself I am being careful.

More problematic are the thoughts that tell me to give up on projects because I am not strong enough to do most jobs alone, to forget about reading books all together because I have trouble concentrating, that talking about what I'm going through makes me boring or needy, that because I've lost friends I'm not capable of being a good one, and that when I'm distracted by pain I cannot expect to have meaningful connections with my community. Running alongside my thoughts about whether or not I should go to the river was this one - *I don't always have energy for long hangouts. That lack of energy makes me no fun to be around.* - and I've got to admit that it is powerful.

I'm understanding this persuasive inner dialog more, and not assigning it so much weight. I'm seeing now, that focusing on avoidance has prioritized my pain, and I'm trying to change that focus. Trying to be a little less careful, a little less afraid. Trying to live more lightheartedly, to push back against my mind's first reaction and all of the black cloud thinking that rolls in after it.

I think now that if I can learn to live with pain well, instead of in tireless opposition to it, I will not have to settle for less than what I want in life. I'm working on living the belief that chronic pain itself doesn't rule things out for me - doesn't hold me back - and that starts with saying yes.

Because, to think I almost missed this: floating in the river, water cooled, splashing and laughing with friends I never see, swimming and using my body, the clearest sky of the summer so far, sun on my skin, being out in nature, breathing deeply... this is the most relaxed I've felt in months, the most connected and undivided, a little bit at peace with myself and my pain.

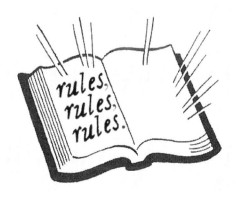

"Time is on our side"

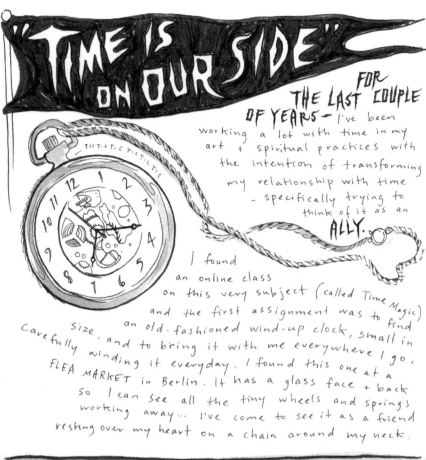

FOR THE LAST COUPLE OF YEARS— I've been working a lot with time in my art + spiritual practices with the intention of transforming my relationship with time — specifically trying to think of it as an **ALLY**.

TIC TIC TIC TIC TIC TIC

I found an online class on this very subject (called Time Magic) and the first assignment was to find an old-fashioned wind-up clock, small in size, and to bring it with me everywhere I go, carefully winding it everyday. I found this one at a FLEA MARKET in Berlin. It has a glass face + back so I can see all the tiny wheels and springs working away... I've come to see it as a friend resting over my heart on a chain around my neck.

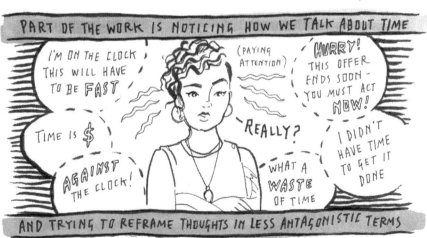

PART OF THE WORK IS NOTICING HOW WE TALK ABOUT TIME

I'M ON THE CLOCK THIS WILL HAVE TO BE FAST

(PAYING ATTENTION)

HURRY! THIS OFFER ENDS SOON— YOU MUST ACT NOW!

TIME IS $

AGAINST THE CLOCK!

REALLY?

WHAT A WASTE OF TIME

I DIDN'T HAVE TIME TO GET IT DONE

AND TRYING TO REFRAME THOUGHTS IN LESS ANTAGONISTIC TERMS

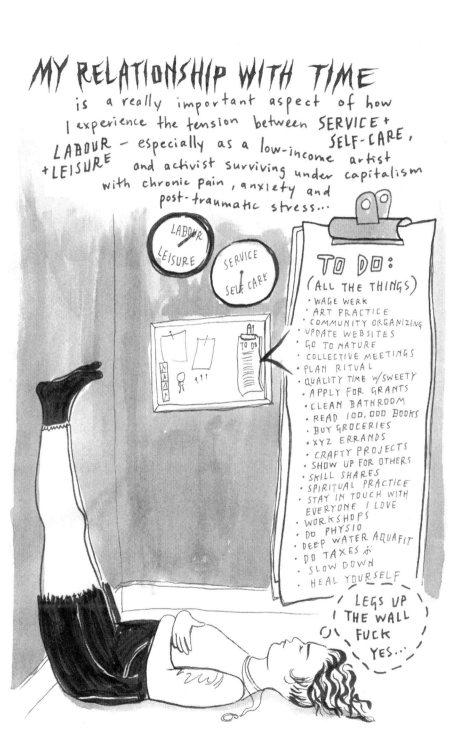

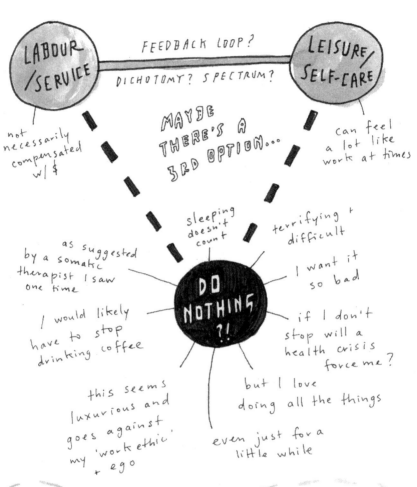

Q: HOW DOES ADDICTION PLAY INTO THE NEED FOR VALIDATION THROUGH PRODUCTIVITY? IS THIS INTERNALIZED CAPITALISM? HOW DO I ENGAGE WITH MY LIMITATIONS IN A COMPASSIONATE WAY AND STILL BE REAL ABOUT THE URGENCY OF THESE TIMES?

A: I DON'T TOTALLY KNOW BUT PART OF THE ANSWER FOR ME LIES IN REMEMBERING THAT TIME IS A COMPLEX, MAGICKAL, OMNI·DIRECTIONAL BEING...

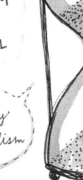

Oh + Destroy Capitalism

OK, YES THAT TOO...

IN THE MEANTIME I AM LEARNING HOW TO:

• consistently follow astrological + lunar cycles + coordinate my own magick endeavors (new moon = chill the fuck out, plant seeds of intention, listen more closely to my body. etc.)

• Take responsibility for how I choose to manage my schedule + not blame Time when I don't do a great job (sorry, Time)

• think of the projects I don't manage to realize as composting + providing nourishing energy for the ones I do get around to

• Pay attention to synchronicity as a way that Time communicates to me that I'm in the right place at the right time and try to co-create these moments more consciously

• Mark the passing seasons w/ ritual and reverence

• TIME TRAVEL * that's another story...

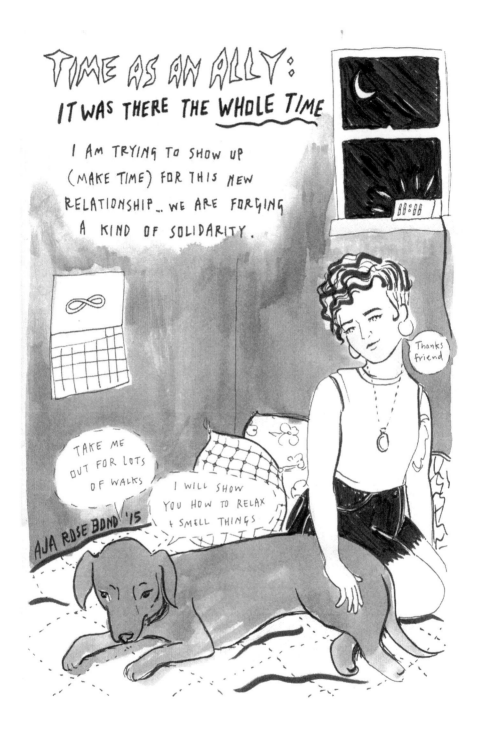

partners in pain

K: I'm Kori. I'm in my late 20's and I have been living with complex medical issues and various amounts of chronic pain since I was a kid. I have a connective tissue disorder that affects my joints, my breathing, my heart and my fatigue levels. I was hit by a car a few years ago, which made my conditions worse and really impacted the ways I have been able to be in relationships. I am a genderqueer trans person, and have experiences dating people in lots of different configurations of genders and orientations. I have also worked in sexual health for a number of years, usually facilitating workshops and producing community radio. I wanted to share some of the things I have learned along the way in hopes that it may offer solidarity to other folks living in bodies in pain. I also hope to provide access to tools so the people who want to date or hook-up with us can do so in ways that take our needs and experiences into consideration.

A: I'm Andi. I'm partnered with Kori and I live with them. I have my own experiences with chronic pain and mental health struggles/resilience. I have almost daily muscle tension that ranges from annoying to debilitating. It is undeniably linked to stress. Oh that pesky mind body connection! That said, I'm writing this article primarily from the perspective of being an ally and caregiver to someone with chronic pain. My perspective on this kind of care is informed by my experiences as a genderqueer white femme who is primarily able-bodied and upper middle classed. I used to be a yoga teacher - which taught me a lot about anatomy and how to take good care of all kinds of bodies. Nowadays I work and play as a youth sex educator, herbalist, witch, photographer, poet, goat walker, and cute-pig-raiser and gardener.

We came to writing this piece as a team, knowing that we are only capable of speaking from our own experiences. We don't speak for everyone, or know what will work for every body. We're sharing with you what works for us - two people who love each other and know each other's bodies well. We both have years of experience in these bodies, learning these skills and (as sex educators) sharing these skills - but that doesn't make us experts, or authorities over anyone's experience. We encourage you to take what works from what we're sharing, and leave the rest. You are the only one in your body - trust that your knowledge is important and valid! We're going to share lots of resources throughout this piece for you to learn more. We hope you can use this piece as a springboard.

K: I think to start this off on the right foot we need to make sure there is a shared understanding of a few big ideas that we are gonna touch back on throughout the article. Firstly CONSENT: much has been written about what consent is and why it's important. *Yes Means Yes* is a great anthology on this topic, if you are looking to learn more.

Understanding ways to integrate good consent practice is something we are going to continue to come back to throughout this piece.

Consent is essentially asking permission before you interact with someone's body. It's being in charge of your own self. It's listening to the other person's response - which should not be coerced. Consent can be revoked at any time for any reason. It's all about trust, communication and being in touch with what feels good in your body.

Secondly, SPOONS: in quick reference terms, it's about knowing your capacity. The concept of spoons, in relation to chronic pain, was coined by Christine Miserandino in her 2003 essay "The Spoon Theory." In our relationship we use phrases like "I don't have the spoons for this right now" or "I'm two spoons too few after walking up that hill" to indicate our energy levels, willingness to do something, or the impact an activity had on either of us.

When consent and spoons come together we have the opportunity to be in tune with the capacities of our bodies and then find ways to communicate that capacity to each other. This all starts with listening to and getting to know your body's limits. When you have an idea of where the limits are you can communicate those limits as boundaries. With good boundaries you can make agreements based on consent.

So for example:

A: *Hey you want to go out for a walk?*

K: *I'm down so long as it's somewhere flat, we walk for less than half an hour and we can stop and have tea somewhere along the way.*

A: *Alright, I'd prefer to walk in nature than in town; can we go to a nature spot that fits within your boundaries?*

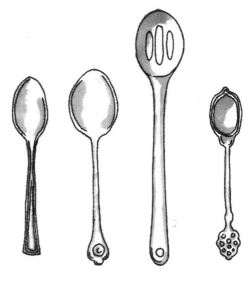

K: *Yeah, I won't be able to bike/walk to there AND walk in nature - can we take the bus or drive to the park?*

A: *Yeah, let's do it.*

A: I think one of the most important parts of making agreements about what we are going to do with our bodies is being able to understand and acknowledge that the expectations we place on what our bodies can do is often unhealthy or unreasonable. Not all bodies can do the same things. We aren't robots. We are taught so often to compare ourselves to others and this often leads us to do things with our bodies that don't actually feel right for us. Learning to understand what your body feels and needs - and accepting those needs and feelings as valid - is extremely important. This learning is something we can do in partnerships and friendships, but it starts and is most important to learn within ourselves first and foremost. You can't be honest with someone else if you aren't honest with yourself first.

As a support person, it's especially important to know that our partners are the experts of their experience. To be a good ally we need to be able to let go of expectations we might have of our partner's bodies, so that we don't shame or guilt them (even unintentionally) into agreeing to something that doesn't really work for their bodies. Being an ally means not only accepting, but celebrating your partner's body, just the way it is.

K: Listening to our bodies, and especially being able to find ways to speak to what feels good or doesn't in our bodies, can be especially challenging when we have had experiences of our bodies being medicalized. Going to doctors appointments and being run through medical tests like x-rays, CT scans, MRIs, having blood taken, having parts of your body measured, manipulated or moved around at the will of doctors, nurses, and radiologists can really mess up one's relationship to bodily autonomy and consent. Lots of times medical professionals really suck at asking if it's ok if they interact with your body, or if something is comfortable or feels ok. We can get used to being poked and prodded without being asked how we feel about it. Ideally medical professionals will have a better "bed-side manner" and find ways to offer you medical attention that doesn't increase pain, anxiety or the feelings of violation that tests and medical procedures can involve. It's hard to learn, or remember, that when we are sharing our bodies with friends, dates and lovers, it is both of our responsibility to ensure that whatever is happening is mutually agreeable.

A: Not every partner we have will be medicalized, or interact frequently with the medical system. When we are in a relationship with someone who has this experience, we may be asked to help or assist them. It's important that this help comes as a request from your partner, not something you force on them when they don't actually want, need or consent to it. Just because someone is in pain, or is sick, doesn't mean they lose the ability to make decisions about what is best for their body. Understanding people with bodies that are sick and in pain to be incapable of making decisions for their own well-being is a belief our society teaches us to hold. Holding onto that belief can create power imbalances in our relationships and leave our partners feeling disempowered and not listened to, which can lead to erosion of trust. Our relationships can stop feeling like partnerships and begin to feel like charity or control, which won't feel good for either partner.

When you are asked to be someone's doctor buddy you'll want to chat with them about what kind of support they are looking for. Do they want you to ask questions? Write notes? Be an emotional support? Speak in the appointment? Not speak? Drive them there, but not attend the meeting? It's important that we respect the boundaries our partner sets and only offer support that is needed and asked for. Same goes when our partner is choosing a course of treatment. We can share our opinions if asked to, or if we ask if it's ok first, but we don't get to make those decisions *for* our partner. When you aren't the person who has to take the medication, eat the special diet, do the daily exercises - you don't get to consent or not consent to the choices.

Pressuring people into healthier life choices, even if done with good intentions, often just leads to feelings of shame and inadequacy in the person you are trying to help. Sure, be honest with the people you love if you see them doing things that are hurting them, but trust them to make the best decisions they can for themselves. Even if they aren't the decisions you would make. You aren't in their body, so you don't make the decisions.

Health looks and feels differently for every person. No one gets to decide for someone else what health or quality of life looks or feels like - even if the other person's choices don't always make sense to us. If it makes sense to them, that is what matters. At the same time, if our partner's choices begin to directly negatively affect us - that's where honest communication and setting boundaries comes in. Not shame, not judgment - just honesty, compassion, curiosity and kindness - for *both* you and your partner.

K: Having a buddy through appointments and routines can be really incredible and helpful. Sometimes the stuff that comes up in a doctor's appointment can be too much to hold alone. Sometimes staying present in appointments can be near impossible. Disassociation can be a *survival mechanism,* one that our bodies engage when navigating difficult procedures and complicated interactions. Having someone advocate for you when you may not be fully present to advocate for yourself is a lifeline. Having another person to help hold what you're going through and help share in building health habits, like stretching, can also be really great. If I don't do some stretching or moving of my body in gentle ways on most days, my pain will get worse. A lot of the time finding motivation to do this type of activity is tricky. Like it's explained in the spoons theory, stretching will make sleeping easier, moving around easier, and it could give me an extra spoon the next day. Doing the stretching may take a spoon and getting down to it, making it actually happen, that can take one too. When I have someone to share in that, it's like doubling up. It's a nice way to spend time with someone I care about, and they are helping me do a thing I need to do to be well in my body. This applies also to food. Sharing in cooking or cleanup can mean a big difference. Sharing tasks may leave me with a bit more capacity in my body to play, make art, make out or get down.

A: Supporting each other in building healthy routines has been really helpful for us. In the morning we wake up, clean the kitchen, make a healthy breakfast, drink coffee or tea, take herbal medicine, read a tarot card each, feed our animals, gather chicken eggs, tend to bone broth, try to move around in our bodies (dancing or stretching), bring in firewood and make a fire. We have these tasks written down on a piece of paper on our fridge and we go through each of them before we turn on our computers or check Facebook.

Doing these things together helps us feel more grounded and well in our bodies. This, in turn, helps our moods, communication and ultimately the quality of our sex life and relationship generally.

As a support person, it's also important to remember that you'll need your own self care routine. For me, that's going to the woods by myself, writing poetry, journaling or reading a book in the bath. I love Kori and I need time away to take care of myself, recharge and get in touch with my needs and feelings. Kori needs this time away from me too - that's why we have separate bedrooms, even though we live together. Sometimes it can be hard to have a clear sense of your needs and boundaries when you are taking care of someone else. For me, cultivating that sense is important and necessary. I have to do it so that I don't burn out, or feel resentful towards Kori because I'm neglecting my own needs. This is true for every relationship, chronic pain or not.

K: So are we ready to talk about sex then?

I am remembering about this relationship I was in right around the same time as my accident. I was dating someone else who had really similar experiences of pain and inflammation in her body. When we would hook up we would often have to stop, take breaks, get pillows to help prop our bodies, change positions, or just cry and laugh together about the bizarre and often painful ways our bodies would collide when we were most excited to be together.

Back then, I hadn't really learned about how to integrate my body's limits into my sex life, especially the new ones I was still mapping out after my accident. Being with someone else who was learning and practicing the same type of thing made space

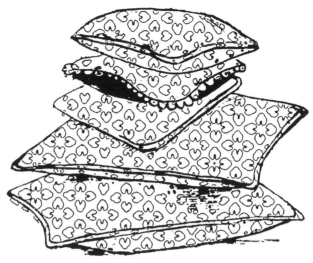

for me to learn more about how to do this well. I have carried the practice of trying to predict my energy levels and communicate desires accordingly. I use checking in throughout sex to let my partners know where I am at, and so I can know what's going on for them. Some times that means we won't get as far as we may have hoped, or that what happens is a modification on what we would want in our dream worlds. There are tools that can be used to help ease the pressure that highly physically demanding interactions, like sex, have on our body.

Using a vibrator on your partner could be useful, as well as things like the Liberator Wedge or specific furniture like the IntimateRider. Modifying toys with handles or straps so that we can utilize the parts of your body that have the most capacity or least pain can be a low cost, DIY project. If hip or back pain makes using a strap-on or having penis-in-vagina sex hard, using a thigh harness or a toy with a handle can give the penetration with less pain in the back.

A: And this brings us back to consent again. For me, consent is just as much about giving permission as it is about getting it. For any relationship - and especially one where folks have chronic pain - it's important to know that what feels good today, might not feel good tomorrow, or even in 5 minutes from now.

What feels good for one body, may not feel good for someone else.

That's why we need to ask - and ask often.

When we have sex we ask lots of questions:

"Does this feel good? No? Ok, what if I do this?"
"Do you have any suggestions?"
"What would feel good to you?"
"How much pressure feels good right now?"
"Can we stop for a minute? I need to put a pillow under my hip."

Taking the time to stop and check in means we learn what feels really good for each other. It makes sex more fun, deep, and connecting. And remember, whatever you partner's answer - *don't take it personally*. If something doesn't feel good it doesn't mean you're bad in bed! It just means it doesn't feel good. Being able to talk about it will allow you to do things that do feel good.

Listening is the skill that is the most important to make you a good lover - trust me on this one.

It's important to take your time and give your partner a chance to take a breath, notice how they feel, really connect to the sensations you are both experiencing. Sometimes this is a quick check in, and sometimes it takes time. Either way it should happen multiple times whenever you are being physically intimate. It may also mean that we don't focus so much on reaching a climax (which isn't possible for everyone's body, or each time they have sex) as we do on treating each other (or ourselves, if we're going at it alone) as sacred, cherished and lovable beings who are worthy of kind touch and support. That support (and what feels hot, sexy, exciting) will look and feel different for each person. Discovering what it looks like for you, or your partner, is all part of the fun!

K: Really good point about giving time for a true check-in. As people in pain we can be given the impression that we are "a burden" when we let people know how much we are actually dealing with. We can downplay our pain levels and try to act more capable than we actually are. Being incapable sucks, it can feel really annoying to be left out of activities you can't participate in, and so sometimes we try and force ourselves to do more than we might actually be ok with. I really appreciate when my partners ask me how I am doing, and encourage me to really ask myself what the true answer is to that question. Sometimes that answer won't be easily expressed with words; it might be easier to explain things as a number (like a pain scale), or using colors or markings (like a pain-map: you can make one on paper, use an app, or even use markers right on your body), or sometimes with growls and grunts.

Usually if my pain levels have reached a point where grunting and growling are the easiest ways to communicate, I am probably past the point where I am going to be able to share my body in intimate and vulnerable ways. It really helps for my partners to know this, so we can make strategies for communicating what we each want, how, where, when, etc.

You know, back to that whole consent thing.

Living in a body that is challenged by pain, mobility issues, medical devices and experiences of medicalization can suck sometimes. It's important to remember that it also gives us a special perspective. Bodies that have learned to live through adversity have built resilience. While there can be a tendency to talk about disAbled bodies in a way that makes them into inspirations (especially to sell products), this is not what I am trying to do here.

I am not happy for the pain I live with, but I am *grateful* for some of the lessons I have learned through living in my disabled body.

Another angle of this that is important to keep in mind, is that being in pain, or having a disability, shouldn't in itself make you less desirable or date-able. People can incorrectly assume that people living in disabled bodies aren't sexual or romantic, or don't want to or can't be in relationships. Don't settle on being with someone who doesn't treat you right, or who isn't someone you want to be with, just because they are willing to be with you and your pain. This is especially true if it seems like there are exploitative dynamics intersecting care-giving and intimate relationships. Some people date people with disabilities in a way that takes advantage of them or exploits power - this is an abusive dynamic.

A: I have never been much for traditional "dating". Personally I think it's kind of boring and unoriginal. I've found it can feel forced *and* it can be really expensive. There's a growing collection of articles online for "crip date ideas". In most of these pieces they recommend focusing on connecting and making dates that feel fun and not too energy intensive for your partner.

If you need to make popcorn and stay in, rather than go out to a movie, that should be not only ok, but encouraged. Taking care of ourselves should be the highest priority in a relationship that is about support and care. There needs to be space for your love (or you) to feel tired, sad, sore, depressed, angry, unable to go outside, unable to go up stairs etc. Without that space we tend to focus constantly on what we are missing, rather than the richness and closeness we can build by being there for each other.

Sometimes this perspective can be hard to take because we live in a society that devalues bodies that are sick or in pain. This is related to a kind of oppression called ableism: the system which empowers certain kinds of bodies over others, and makes access to spaces, places, experiences and resources more challenging for some people than others. We *can all learn* to understand, unpack and challenge ableism in ourselves, our relationships and the world. There's tons of great resources and projects that you can access online to learn more.

K: Obviously your experiences are going to be as unique as you are. Our bodies, abilities and capacities can and do all change over time. We hope that you are able to take this information and the resources we've included and put them to use in ways that feel suitable for your life. We wish you experiences of support, fulfillment, passion and love.

Remember - you don't deserve anything less.

Meredith Butner

in between days

I didn't do a single thing today that resembles self care. I'm feeling depressed, heavy, and blank. Even though gas is a million bucks a gallon I went for a drive blasting mid-90s hardcore and The Mountain Goats. I rolled down the windows and sang along loudly. I broke the speed limit and let myself feel the blur of things passing by, let the wind tangle my hair.

There is something bugging me I haven't been able to put into words, something I thought a car ride might fix. Speed to satisfy a need for motion, forward momentum I can't otherwise grab hold of.

I've been living an in between kind of life, somewhere along the drawn-out road from injury to recovery. My pain remains chronic and characteristically unpredictable, but there is comfort in distance from the urgency and emergency that dismantled my healthy house. When asked if my back is getting better, I'll always answer "slowly" - confident that I am moving forward, but inching along at a pace I mostly cannot see.

Life here feels really challenging. I have a long way to go, but struggle with motivation. It seems so odd; months ago the mere presence of pain was enough to send me spinning out desperately in all directions; visiting a set of doctors who would run tests and document my injury to fulfill paperwork obligations for my employer, while actively exploring the sea of alternative options, searching for treatment I could connect with when I'd been let down by injections and surgery before. I did these things like a reflex response, with energy despite the exhaustion of the experience, until my injury brought me to a complete stop.

For a time pain halted my body, restricting my ability to move. For more than three weeks, at its most acute, I couldn't leave the second floor of my house. I struggled to assemble myself into a vertical position, barely able to manage the crooked shuffle from my bedroom to the bathroom. My meals and pills appeared, attached to hope and worry from the hearts that brought them up to me - husband, housemates, and friends. I napped when pain meds permitted me an hour or two of relief and played music through headphones to distract my senses when the lights were out but my body couldn't rest.

Of all of the adjustments pain has insisted from me throughout the course of this injury, accepting myself in that place of vulnerability was the hardest thing I've had to do. I felt, on the one hand, absolutely without control, unfastened in the drifts of pain, too weak and tired to long for my old life and, on the other hand, resisting. I stuck stubbornly to the one assertion I was able to make - *I will not go to the hospital* - then gave myself over to pain in a way I never had before. I was forced to see that being pain-free wasn't a decision I could just make; there was a process my body needed to go through and, at that moment, it demanded to be still.

When the pain subsided a bit and my head felt clearer, I collected my hopes around things that I had had positive experiences with in the past: visits to my physical therapy and chiropractic appointments, heat and ice treatments, consistent meals of anti-inflammatory foods, support from supplements and herbs, and regular swimming, stretching and relaxation exercises. I did these things as I was able to, and little by little I felt myself getting stronger.

I remember my first day back to the gym after weeks of being absent. My husband had helped me change into my swimsuit at home and I was wearing it under my clothes as I labored across the main space, a room full of weight machines and healthy, sweating bodies, towards the locker room and pool. I remember the way I struggled to remove my shoes and place them in a locker, and the true effort behind each motion leading me closer to the water. That day I mostly just floated, walked and kicked in the pool, let the water loosen and stretch me with its altered gravity, but half of a year later I was swimming 40 minutes of laps five days a week and the journey from the door of the gym, through the locker room, to the pool was uncomplicated.

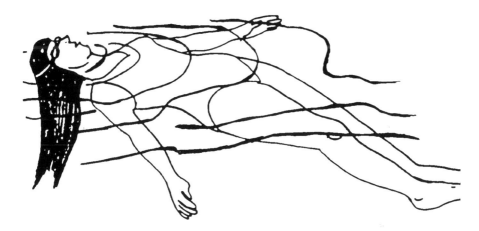

As my pain moved out of the acute phase, managing it became a lot more subtle. Something I find endlessly frustrating about pain that is chronic is that there isn't always a direct connection between an action, movement, or activity and a pain response. Over the long term, in my experience, cause and effect became more tenuous, less easy to decipher. The new normal for my life includes pain, without a level of urgency. Things have stabilized - I can work part-time again, I can sit at a table for a meal or a meeting, I take on projects and can join friends for small hangouts and adventures - and with that stability comes a loss of context for everyday choices that seems to put my motivation at risk.

At some point along the way, the daily commitment I need to make to self-care has become overwhelming. I have seen and felt the cumulative results of sticking to what I know works but, for all the effort my healthy routine requires, the pay off comes so small and slow. When I count up the supplements, measure out the tinctures drop by drop, add up the minutes I need to give to exercise, treatment, rest, and cooking daily just to, hopefully, feel decent... my head spins a little. Sometimes trading swimming for time with friends, or meal planning for comfort food seems more immediately do-able day to day. Sometimes slacking, and the easy distraction of DVRed television feels like a necessary diversion. I can certainly find the argument to allow myself this kind of leisure, but it quickly becomes a slippery slope. A pattern starts, choosing comfort over health, and my mood and confident determination drops as the pain levels creep back up.

There are also days when I go into hiding, when just brushing my hair seems like too huge a task to muster. It isn't so much the pain itself I can't feel my way through on days like this, but recognizing the whole *experience* of pain and what it demands in response, how it emotionally depletes me. In a way pain has become like weather around me, the storm in which I operate.

I recently came across the following poem by the writer anais nin:

Risk

And then the day
came,
when the risk
to remain
tight
in a bud
was more
painful
than the risk
it took
to Blossom.

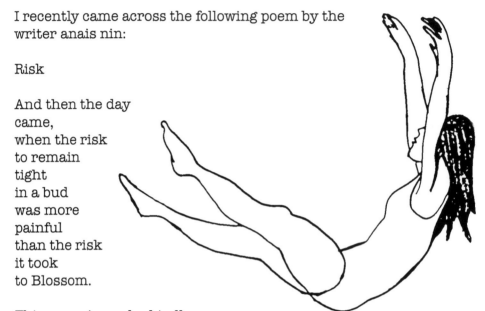

This poem is, undoubtedly,
relatable to a wide variety of situations, but the words struck me as important right now because much of my experience with chronic pain has been a struggle of calculating risks and negotiating trade-offs. Some days it does seem more comfortable to stagnate in injury than to deal with the fierce commitment it takes to pursue a healing that is unpredictable. It surprises me how easily I've slipped into this space that is supposed to be transitional, pulled up protection like covers around me to hide out from the exhaustion and heartbreak of chasing a recovery that isn't guaranteed. To move toward health with an increased intentionally is to make yourself vulnerable to a whole world of things beyond your control - a big risk for sure - but roll down the windows, turn up the stereo, it's probably a car ride worth taking.

Noemi Martinez

earth moves slowly beneath us as we wait

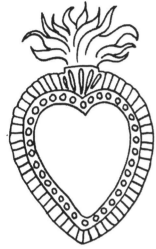

waiting at clinic.
man snoring softly
next to me.
pay $35 upfront.
Can you make a payment
on your balance?

Sit, wait.
Man snores.
Check email on phone.
Check email on phone.
Read Terabithia
Read Norma Cantu.
Sit, wait.
Check email on phone.
Return email to Lina,
Re: location of panteon.
Sit, wait, clouds form.
Looks like rain.

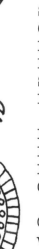

Read Emmy's poems.
Envious, lovely forms.
Man snores.
Check email on phone.

Quiet coughing spell
with cough drops
gifted by my mom
before she left us,
left the valley for
colder seasons.
Snow, trees.
Consider leaving.
Have already paid

$25 upfront.
Entered a payment plan
for enormous balance
of allergy tests
insurance didn't cover.
Who knew?
Sit, Wait.
"¿Tiene cita?"
"¿Que doctor quiere ver?"
¿Tiene seguro?

Additional parking
in rear.
laugh at joke.

2 t.v.s on.
one is english soap opera
with volume turned down.
other is spanish
morning today style show
turned up
we are glued.

Wait.
Man is called.
Lunch hour is over.
Doctors return.
Think twice
about being here.
I've already paid.

Finish chapbook.
Check email on phone.
Check email on phone.
Text sister,
babysit on Friday?

Will tell Dr.
of insurance change.
So MRI's and cat scans
and sleep studies a go.

at affordable prices
with payment plans.

hope she doesn't
get mad
i haven't done
them yet.

wait,sit,wait.
Man with cane shuffles in.
A Señora with another Señora
walk in.
"aqui traigo a mi comadre
Ya no ve"

Check email on phone.
think of music.
think of poems.
think of poems
in text form.
think of devils
and twenty dollar bills.

Check email on phone.
Sip water,
parched painful.
they call my name.
nurse says
"dr says she knows
whats wrong with you
again."
so predictable, I am.
yes, on throat, yes
on sinuses.
Nurse hands me
allergy results,
he says
no more mangoes
no more bananas
he says
start eating meat again.
he doesn't know

my heart is
allergic to eating blood
(yes, trauma dramatic
induced by 100.1 fever)
Dr. Mbeki walks in
touches my knee
sorry to be late.

i tell her of exams
she says its pap smear
time, save myself -
i'm bleeding.
RX for throat, nose, head.
I think she likes me
maybe one day
I'll tell her everything

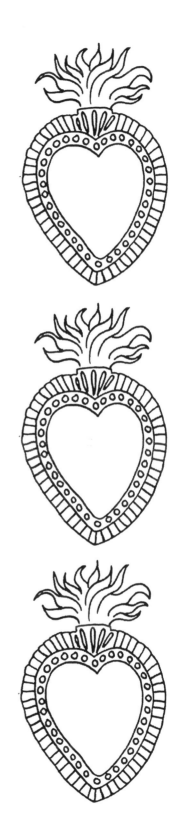

fake it till you make it

When I was 19, my therapist was a young German woman on her way to getting certified as a Jungian analyst. Once a week I went to her office in the West Village in the hopes that she could help me out of my severe depression. It seems in hindsight like it was winter for the entire 9 months I lived in New York; all my memories are of grey concrete and icy wind, slushy subway steps and sunset at 4 pm. Everything I did during that time I did on automatic, like a robot. If I hadn't had my nanny job to get me out of my studio apartment 5 days a week I probably would never have gone outside. Whereas an accomplishment for me before the depression might include working in a collective or writing a short story, now it meant getting myself fed and dressed every day. And of course, going to see my therapist Frauke every week.

In one such session with Frauke the topic of my spirituality arose. I had been a very spiritual child. Not religious, although I was raised Catholic and went to church most every Sunday for the first 15 years of my life. My spirituality was something I was born with and nurtured through my play, through dance and through reading. I had my own beliefs and rituals that did not come from my family or community but that I practiced on my own. The things I knew and felt changed as I grew but were never absent from my heart. Not until I hit that depression.

Often when people try to distinguish between depression and other dark states of being such as grief, they note that depression is not an excess of feeling but a lack of it. It is the inability to connect with oneself and with the world. From my own experience of depression I would agree and I would say that when I was depressed I also lost the ability to connect with the spirit world. I no longer had an innate sense of my spirituality. When I looked inside myself my inner world had gone from 3 to 2 dimensions, a flat image with no horizons. If I tried to grasp at a feeling or belief, it turned to vapor and floated out of my reach.

So one day, I found myself telling Frauke about my total disconnection from my former spirituality.

"I can't feel or believe in anything anymore," I said in our session. Frauke acknowledged the depth of this loss, and then she said to me,

"You don't believe right now I can hold this belief for you. I will believe for you until you can believe again."

I found her response extremely comforting and it has stayed with me ever since. I have often used this phrase in other ways with people I was supporting through a struggle, perhaps letting a friend who felt hopeless know that I could feel that hope for them until they were able to feel it again themselves. What I learned from that part of my life was a sort of "fake it till you make it" tactic for surviving an extremely dark time. The sort of time in which all the laws you have previously lived by do not apply any more, and there is nothing to anchor you to the earth. I was going through the motions of a lot of things, without really connecting to them. That meant brushing my teeth. It meant going out with someone to a museum. It meant reading a book. I believe that, while I couldn't FEEL the benefit of those actions as I performed them, they contributed to my eventual resurfacing from the depression. My spiritual self, too, lay dormant. But I let Frauke hold it for me until I began to thaw. Then it was there for me stronger than before.

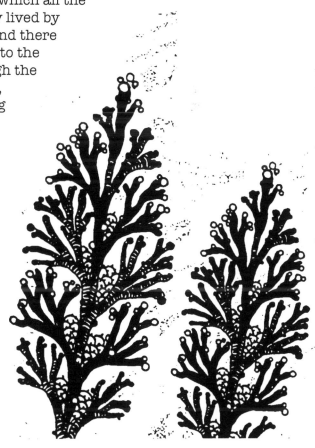

When I developed chronic back and pelvic pain, there were a lot of parallels to that earlier time of darkness. Mostly this is because I sank into a serious grief and depression as my condition worsened with no promise of an eventual recovery. The numbness, the inability to connect to every day life and the things that sustain me, returned. Additionally, I was on a lot of pain meds that dulled my senses. And the pain caused me to check out of my body in order to endure it. My birthday, that first year I developed chronic pain, I just sat in my chair at my party in a haze of pain and narcotics. I watched the proceedings from a distance, unable to feel the sunshine, taste the food or bond with friends. During this crisis time at the onset of my illness, I felt even more estranged from myself than I had during my depression at age 19.

Maybe because I had developed such a powerful toolkit during my previous hardship, I charged full force into the care of this new condition. In spite of how checked out I felt, I advocated strongly for my needs and sought out information and healing with drive. It was drive, but I was definitely on automatic. Some part of me believed that I needed to do these things to take care of myself, but I did not feel hope or passion about them. Quite the opposite: with the help of a bureaucratic health care system that seemed to delight in throwing obstacles in my path, I mostly felt extreme hopelessness. And just like when I was 19, my sense of the sacred was painfully absent. This crucial aspect of my sense of wholeness and well being had absconded once again.

So, I found myself a second time in the position of going through the motions. In some ways, it was easier because I had the success of that last time to remind me that it is possible to come out on the other side of seemingly endless crisis. I think that's part of what motivated my self-advocacy, which included a search for spiritual healing.

The problem with a spirituality that has not been cultivated by the family or the community is that a practice is not passed on.

I made my practice up as I went, but there was little concrete to hold onto when times got tough. I didn't know what resonated with me a lot of the time. Trying to find what felt right when I was depressed and checked-out was even more difficult. I ended up testing a number of different methods of healing and spiritual practice and coming as close as I could to something that felt right.

One of the first things I did was get energy work from, surprisingly, an MD who worked in the chronic pain clinic at my hospital. He was a nice old man who'd primarily worked with veterans, and who did all the allopathic stuff but believed in energy and crystal healing as well. I also worked for a time with a witch who helped me develop a strong visualization ritual. I saw a talk therapist and later a movement therapist as well. I studied curanderismo on my own time.

None of these things made my pain go away. And none of them were powerful enough that I felt a full revival of my connection to my spirituality. But I did them anyway. I ended up taking bits and pieces from each practice and making my own that primarily consisted of a series of rituals I performed in front of my altar nightly. I had actual physical exercises I did with my body (from physical therapy), and a series of visualizations, as well as tasks like lighting the candles on my altar. I did them dutifully every night for months and months. Sometimes I found them soothing, other times I found them hollow and could barely get myself to try. Sometimes my practice of these rituals was purely fueled by rage. But I did them, and I kept going to my many appointments with various healers as well. I kept getting out of bed and going to work and buying groceries and everything else that was daily life.

You don't wake up one day and suddenly have it back. You're not suddenly past the crisis. You don't suddenly feel Good and Alive again. It happens very slowly, and it's not a straight line but a series of ups and downs where the ups reach a little higher than the downs go low.

All that year and more one of my close friends had been struggling with the suicide of a loved one. It was remarkable how similar our experiences of grief and depression were during that whole period of time. She'd call me on the phone crying and the words coming out of her mouth sounded like the thoughts running through my own head. When I saw her beginning to have days that were a little better, I saw that I was also beginning to have those days. A day when gravity was back for awhile and we could feel the dirt under our toes. A day when we could laugh from somewhere deeper than our skin. That day would end and then the next might be another difficult one. But eventually the crisis passed into something more like maintenance, and it wasn't such a chore anymore, it wasn't just going through the motions. I didn't just have to believe, I could feel it again.

It's funny how I practice my series of rituals less now that I'm past the crisis time of my chronic pain. I don't have to be so rigorous anymore, because I feel connected to it moment to moment. I do however want to cultivate my practice more thoughtfully and concretely, so it's there at full strength whenever I might need it again. I also want to share some of these practices with a larger community, because I feel that the strength and consistency of a group could have sustained me in even more effective ways. I want to be able to pass on to my future child a meaningful and open-ended practice that she doesn't have to invent totally from scratch when she encounters hardship. I know, at the least, that I will be there for my child during those dark times to say exactly what my therapist said to me: I will hold this for you until you are able to hold it yourself again.

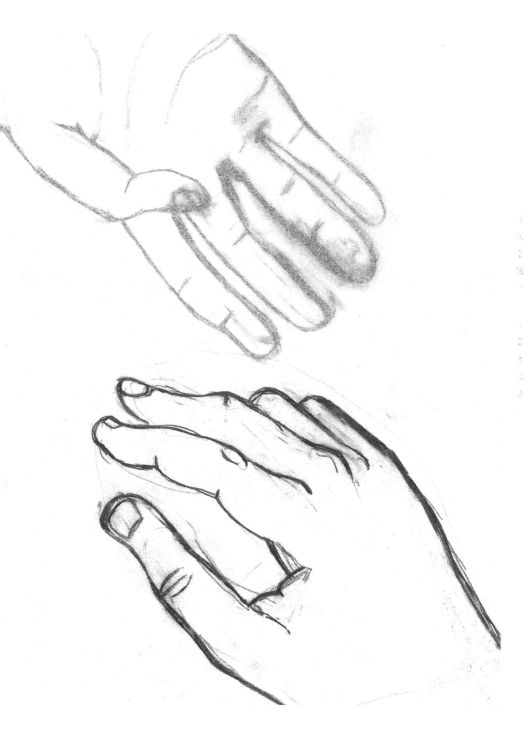

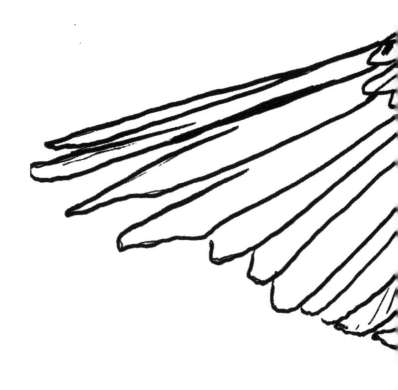

on support

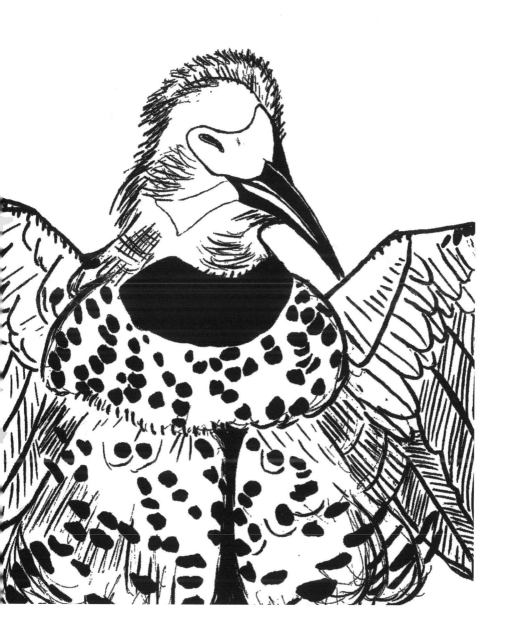

a discussion of
chronic pain, support, lacking support, radical culture, and life.

Illness. If I grew up believing the doctors always did what was best for their patients, I knew that was utter nonsense by the time I was 21. My mother almost died that summer, after her surgeon botched an operation. Before the medical staff knew about the leakage they released her home. During the two days following her visit she became paranoid - calling friends to explain how her family was out to get her, and increasingly treating us all with intense suspicion. As the pain increased my father and I put her in the car and began a long, painful and exhausting drive back to New York City. Hours later we found out that had she not returned she could've died: the surgeon botched the operation, punctured a hole, and left her leaking spinal fluid.

There've been many scares, of ranging intensity, since 1998, when my mother was diagnosed with Reflex Sympathetic Dystrophy (RSD). RSD is a neurological syndrome that creates a deep burning sensation and intense and consistent pain which those who suffer struggle to describe. It often spreads throughout different regions of the body. While there is likely a genetic pre-disposition to the disorder, it takes a trauma of some sort to push it into motion. In my mother's case it was most likely a surgery on her knee that a doctor botched - after which he fudged her records to evade responsibility.

On an everyday level the disorder takes over - the pain increases, leading to more treatments and more medications, and then leading to more doctor appointments. Sometimes the treatments work, and sometimes they don't. Sometimes they work the first time but less so over the long-term. And things have gotten better from their worst: my mother doesn't require a wheelchair anymore, the doctors actually believe she has the illness she has, and sometimes her pain level is manageable.

But she lives the pain on an everyday basis, which means that "better" is relative to the height of the severity of her pain, not to the point when she had no pain at all. She lives in between doctor appointments - each of which offers either no news, or good news, or bad news, or more waiting for test results. It's an ongoing process of waiting. And there's multiple appointments every week. She assuages her pain through the use of a variety medications that have any number of side effects. A complete list of the ways that the pain she suffers from affects her daily life would go on much longer.

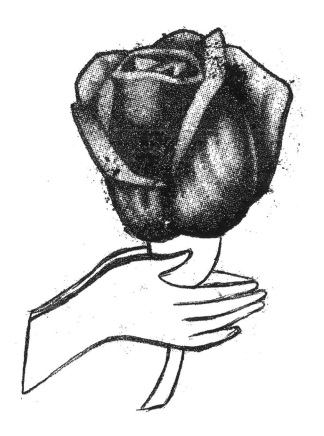

Contextual Complications. While the physical pain ebbs and flows - though never subsides - there's the stress caused by all the other factors that come with illness under neoliberal capitalism. Because of my father's job, where he works under a serious degree of stress, my mother is able to have private insurance. But the insurance companies, like much of the medical industry, function under a near state of impunity. Talking to people with severe, long-term illness in the U.S. can be as heart-wrenching an experience as hearing torture stories - because, realistically, the insurance companies engage in what can only be called campaigns of harassment, if not terror, against patients with pain disorders. This commonly happens through challenges to test and medication coverage, limitations on what doctors the patient is able to see, and the painful and disempowering bureaucratic processes that the companies rely on to fill their records and concretize patient disempowerment.

In my mother's case, on various occasions, they've simply cut-off the drugs she uses to relieve the pain - leaving my parents to load up credit cards and go through hard and sordid processes of State bureaucracy to push the insurance company to live up to their responsibility of covering her medications. The struggles with the insurance company leave her, and my family, in a state of fear and insecurity about what happens next. Such fear has pervasive ramifications on physical, emotional and interpersonal levels for everyone involved.

Lawyers don't like to pick up RSD cases - they're known for being anomalously hard to prove in court. My parents search and they get excited that maybe they've found someone, and then it doesn't happen. The lawyer won't take the case.

Waged labor is a particularly complex issue for individuals suffering with a pain disorder, and this is certainly the case for my mother. I grew up in a working class family, and over the years my parents were able to ground themselves a little more. By the time of my teens my mother was able to go through college, and by the last year of my teens they were able to afford a house. One of my mother's proudest moments was when she finished her Social Work degree. She was able to work for a year. But between the multiple doctor appointments each week, the effects of the drugs she needs to take, the disempowerment of her situation, as well as other factors, she faces a consistent reality of being unwaged. In my mother's case, she is incredible at her work: as a woman who experienced poverty and hardship in many ways, her heart intertwines with her technical skill and empathetic abilities to be an anomalously positive exception in a field of exhausted, overworked, and often-times insensitive professional social mediators. With the situation she is in, however, she's been unable to practice her skill for sometime, leading to another sort of pain that is deeply frustrating and hard to cope with.

Support over the Long-Term. Long-term support work for someone undergoing a long-term non-terminal illness that thoroughly injures their ability to live a normal life means that much of the time lives collide. Support work over the long-term for a non-terminal illness means that multiple people need to live their lives while taking the particular circumstances of the person facing illness into account. Career, desire, responsibility to others aside from the person facing illness, the need to be personally happy - all of these need to be taken into account both for and from the person facing illness and those being support of them.

On questions of support I think there are two major things to remember:

(1) Severe and long-term illness is pervasive: it not only affects the person facing illness, but also those in close relation to them. In my family's case it's meant living in an environment that is often unstable and dealing with fear that exacerbates - sometimes severely - other life stresses. It has also meant engaging in and developing problematic coping mechanisms. That the main factor is out of anyone's control leads to a sense of long-term frustration that results from an inherently disempowering situation - since the illness wasn't a choice, there's a constant feeling of injustice.

(2) Long-term support through illness requires adjusting multiple lives to a situation that is out of the control of any individual involved. Since multiple lives are impacted, negotiating needs and desires while also being

responsive and responsibly supportive requires serious intentionality and effort.

Long-term support work means acknowledging that we exist in social webs: regardless of what capitalist fantasy tries to push, none of us are isolated individuals. Almost everyone exists within some sort of tangible community, and most of us simultaneously exist in various tangible communities at one time. These communities compose our social webs - and within communities that are intentionally supportive and resistant to capitalist atomization, the threads of care that compose the webs are thicker. But regardless of the stated or implied intention of a given community, being supportive to a person coping with a chronic pain disorder, or any other long-term pervasive illness, means that we test the strength of these webs.

It's helpful to assess social webs when engaging in long-term support efforts, and to be up front about the situations that exist. The unfortunate reality is that much of the time illness is something people don't talk about, something we don't ask those struggling through it about, and something we don't discuss with someone supporting another person through. In my experience, and that of others I know, those supporting a person facing illness also need to have solid bases of support: supporters need to be supported if they're to maintain their own health and be adequately supportive of the person facing illness.

I've often times failed in trying to be supportive of my mother and my family. By "failed" I mean that many times I've avoided being pro-actively helpful, I've mis-prioritized, and I've not fairly dialogued with my mother or my father regarding their needs. Sometimes instead of having the necessary dialogues, I've simply evaded them, which has meant that my mother and my family have dealt with lacking support where it may have been necessary. While I struggle with an immense amount of guilt over my actions, what my mother lives with - the pain she faces, the feeling of being inadequately supported, and the isolation of it all - is something she can't escape. I've found that important to remember.

And many other times I have had these dialogues and it's made an impact on the ability of my mother to cope with the pain and complications she faces; it's also helped the rest of my family. During these I've been helpfully supportive by providing tangible forms of assistance: an ear to listen and a shoulder to cry on, rides to the hospital, coming back to my parents home from far away to provide a necessary presence, and so on. Sometimes these dialogues are utterly painful, and since there's no easy answers, the dialogues don't yield exciting options. That's the reality of these sorts of situations.

Acknowledging fuck-ups in dealing with support work doesn't mean that you've simultaneously, or even consequentially, changed behavior patterns - actually changing behavior patterns is the only thing that accomplishes that effect, and that's much harder than acknowledgment. And long-term support work means you fuck up a lot. As a participant in radical movement building, as a participant in transient cultures like punk and DIY, and as a student and worker living in an economy that imposes intense conditions of precarity on the working class, the negotiations I've had with my parents have been particularly complicated by time, choice and distance. My life choices have directly affected what kind of support I give.

Within the cultures of resistance that I've participated in - largely explicitly anti-capitalist and DIY oriented-issues of illness and support over the long-term are not at the core of political practice (thankfully, this is not the case in all radical cultures - one here thinks of organizations like ACT UP amongst other examples where support work has been crucial). Realistically, it's often the case that many anti-capitalists and DIY participants evade the subjects of illness and support work. In my experience we need these types of discussions to be open and core to our projects if we hope to provide safe spaces that create substantial relations of mutual aid that tangibly help participants. It's been the rare exception that I've been able to feel that issues of support and illness are crucial subjects of discussion and action within these cultures of resistance. And while urgent or immediate situations within and outside of radical circles are often able to garner immediate support - long-term support efforts are a very different experience. Long-term support efforts mean ongoing intentionality and struggle that short-term efforts may not.

In conclusion, it's important to remember that within social webs the person facing illness is someone you love - which means that they need you, and you need them. Illness is a burden to the person facing it, but they are not their illness. Perhaps this is one of the most important things to remember. Support efforts mean treating the person facing the illness as the person they are in all their totality - they are facing illness, but that's only one of many aspects of them. What's important is integrating their needs into your relation with them, and vice versa.

In my case, my mother is someone I'm truly fortunate to have a close relationship with, and my biological family unit is a crucial part of my life. I simply wouldn't be who I am in my life without the care and love they've given me, which illustrates all the more usefully the social web I am in. I want to be supportive of them because of my feeling of overwhelming love, not simply my responsibility (which is also there). I want my mother and my family to know that I'm there, and I want my mother to live a life that is fulfilling and happy. I have a role in that. And I fuck-up. Grappling with the guilt and fuck-up's and changing behaviors to make better choices, and thus provide more adequate support, has been a major struggle - and it's a struggle that has been hard for my family to deal with. But it's a necessary and on-going process in this sort of situation.

Note: I have left this piece as it was originally published in 2008. If written today I would write some of it differently. Most importantly, I would give more attention to incredible strength that my mother has maintained in the years she has struggled with a series of painful and traumatic medical issues that no one should have to endure. And I would attend more to the importance of love, carefulness and understanding in supportive relationships.

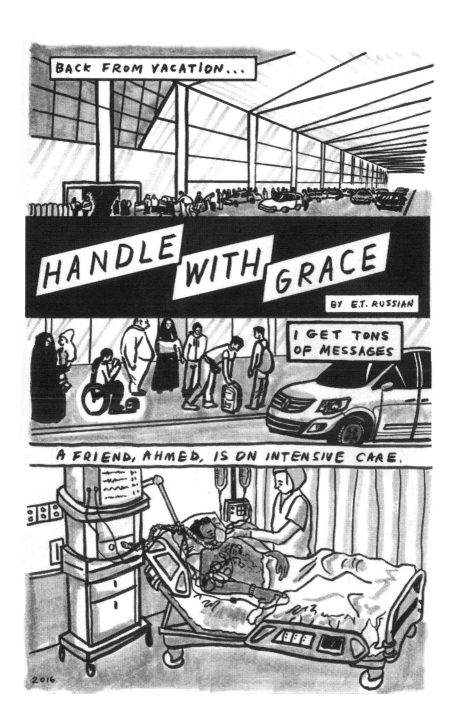

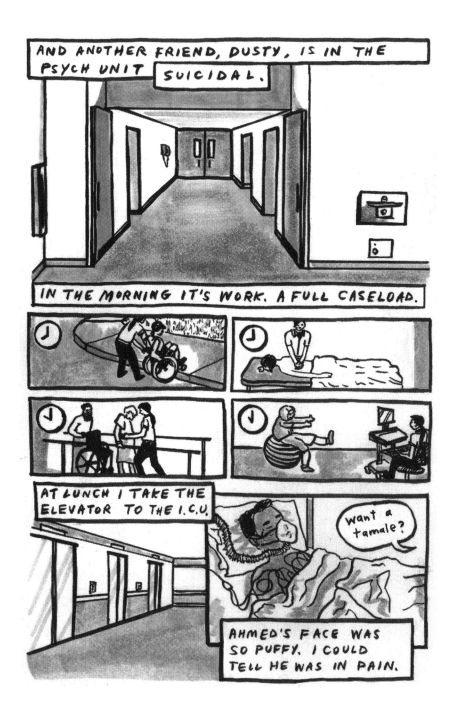

BACK AT WORK...

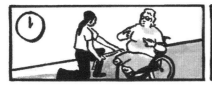
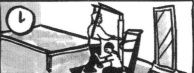
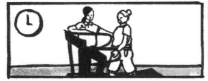
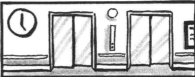

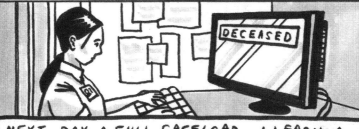

NEXT DAY A FULL CASELOAD. I LEARN A
CLIENT HAS DIED. SHE HAD CANCER AND
A.L.S. SHE REQUESTED DEATH WITH DIGNITY.

AFTER WORK...

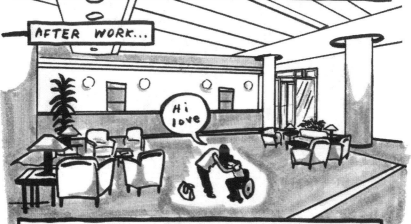

I MEET INDIRA IN THE LOBBY OF DUSTY'S
PSYCH UNIT ACROSS TOWN.

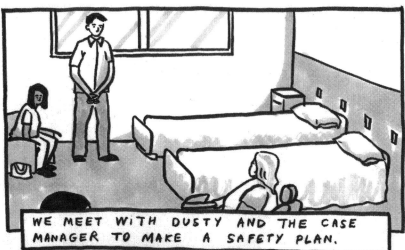

WE MEET WITH DUSTY AND THE CASE MANAGER TO MAKE A SAFETY PLAN.

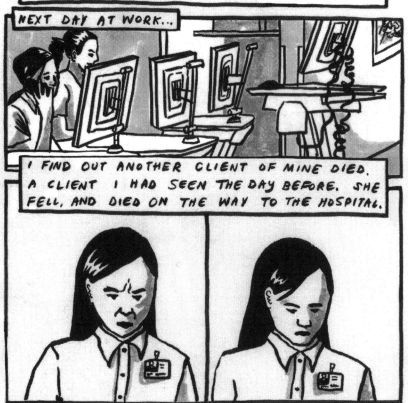

NEXT DAY AT WORK...

I FIND OUT ANOTHER CLIENT OF MINE DIED. A CLIENT I HAD SEEN THE DAY BEFORE. SHE FELL, AND DIED ON THE WAY TO THE HOSPITAL.

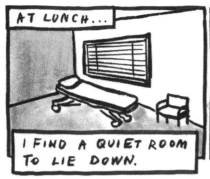

AT LUNCH...

I FIND A QUIET ROOM TO LIE DOWN.

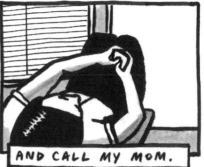

AND CALL MY MOM.

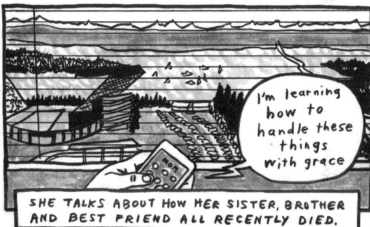

I'm learning how to handle these things with grace

SHE TALKS ABOUT HOW HER SISTER, BROTHER AND BEST FRIEND ALL RECENTLY DIED.

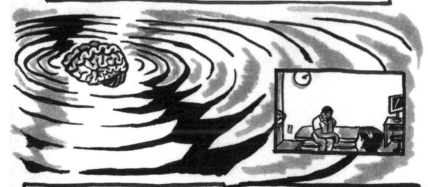

MY MIND SWIMMING, I TELL MYSELF "JUST TWO MORE CLIENTS."

THEN, MY LAST CLIENT OF THE DAY REPORTS HE IS SUICIDAL.

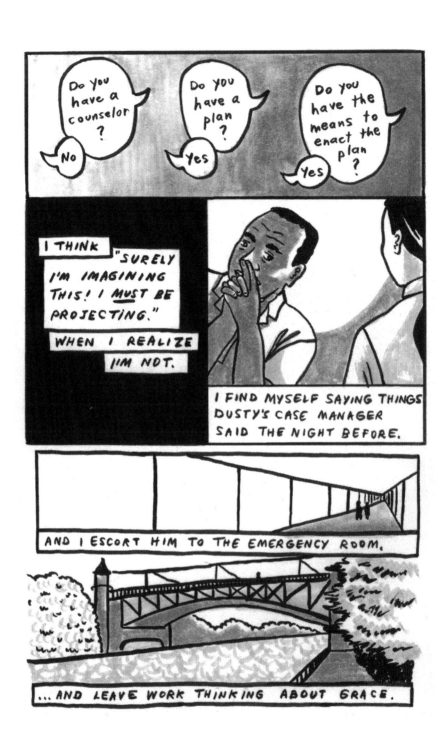

Jonah Aline Daniel

private ocean

I have experienced pain and illness over the past several years
as a descent into a private ocean
Many things filter down through the layers of vegetation and wildlife
Some crash repeatedly on the shore
Some are swept by invisible and unpredictable currents, long lost
It's a world of depth and vastness,
wildness and stillness both
Touch and smell are different here and so is the light
Some things make it through the layers, some disintegrate,
some become bloated or distorted,
some break apart into fragments,
smashed against rocks and reefs
Words are different here too-
all shapes and vibration
More like touch than sound

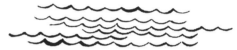

I live more and more above the water these days
Taking my oxygen, my meals on dry land,
feet on the ground, body upright
I meet you here, close to the surface
But the depths remain,
the currents and the tides, they call to me.
I feel their pull.
I listen carefully, with every cell
I learn to give these depths voice,
to respond to their pull without being submerged
I will never abandon you I say
and yes, of course, I will return

And what do I need from others?
I need people to pay attention
Not overextend beyond their own comfort or boundaries
Not make a big deal, but be in relationship in a way that is attentive
Responsive

And I need to not be above water all the time to have human connection
To know that I can be deep in my own process of sensation and
self responsiveness and still be desired,
still be loved,
still be hot or fun or interesting
To know that my wisdom and my depth are valued,
even if I can't walk fast or run ever or remember everything or hold my body
up or keep my eyes open
And I'm still learning how to ask.

sick

Fifteen years ago, the person I love the most got sick. I was living in a punk house, she was in school. At first it was emergency mode, of course. Get her away from the family. Figure out what these drugs were the doctor gave her. She came out to live with me and we poured over medical books and drug books, trying to decipher the insane medical language.

I think I had an idea that we could fix it. I thought the problems were environmental, that the doctors were crazy. It thought we could fix it by diet and maybe environment. In the beginning, it seemed to take up my life, but the truth was, I don't think I spent that much time actually doing anything. I mean, we must have only spent a few hours a few times trying to decipher the books, and I don't remember cooking that much in the stupid house we lived in. It is that trap of emergency mode. You feel like you're doing a lot when it's really your body stress and brain crazy.

I remember then, feeling angry. Angry that there was nothing I could do. Angry at the world for making this happen to her. And angry at all the old angers too - the angers about having to take care of my mom and my dad, of never getting to have an easy time, of no one ever taking care of me, of the stupid fucks and stupid jobs and no community. We were in a new town; we didn't have much in the way of friends. The anger and helplessness made me self-absorbed. I thought about her all the time, I was absorbed by how I felt about her, but I was not there for her. We've talked about it and she's said that even if I wasn't there, actually, she still knew I was there for her in my heart, but I am still ashamed by it. And I think this is something that happens a lot. I have seen it in other places. And I think it's important to talk about and recognize and maybe then it can be avoided.

I see the crisis/anger thing happen a lot - like when my friend Hanna's boyfriend got in an accident and had bleeding in his brain and was in the hospital for weeks and all the friends came and swarmed the place. Crisis. Would he live? Would he be permanently damaged? Everyone was there, trying to give support, freaking out. But it was too much, and Hanna just wanted some quiet, she didn't want to have to deal with everyone else's shit, everyone else's memories and drunkenness and fear.

"Go away, go away,' she said 'I'm going to be the one taking care of him."

And the friends got pissed. At her, maybe at their own things too. Blame, self blame. And when the bleeding finally stopped and he had to relearn movement and speech in the rehab hospital for months, the friends were mostly so angry or alienated they didn't come to help much. Burned out. But that was when it was really needed, and really mattered.

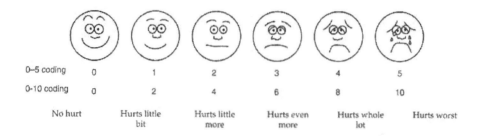

Caregiving is something about pacing. And I don't mean, "take care of yourself first." I think that is bullshit. but it is about learning to caregive yourself while learning to caregive others. It is about getting out of savior mode into something that is workable, and recognizing that this is long term and needs will change: my needs and hers. Sometimes I'll find something that seems workable like I'll decide to cook breakfast for her every morning, and then it becomes unworkable. It starts to feel like a burden, and then I get resentful, but the truth is, she doesn't care one way or the other if I cook her breakfast every morning. And one of the big problems with the whole burden/resent thing is that if I'm already feeling burdened by things she's not even asking me to do, then there's not as much of a chance that she's going to ask me for the things she really needs. Plus, feeling like a burden sucks. I know. So it's being aware of things like that, and being flexible. Finding the small things that actually do matter and that are doable, and then being flexible with the extra stuff. And knowing that some weeks I'll be more present and capable than other weeks. For me, a big thing has been to stop promising to do things I won't be able to do.

One thing I had to do was to learn to recognize her new body language. Her face sometimes looks like it's saying "get the hell away from me," when it is really saying "I feel like I'm going to puke." The pain movements sometimes look like "leave me alone" when it's really just hurt. I've had to learn to not take things so personally. I've had to accept that she is in pain and sick, and to take that in to consideration not just in my mind but in my body too. To feel the weight of it and the sadness of it and breathe and move forward. I have to cry. I have to have other people to talk with. I have to mourn. I have to be angry at the world and the people who have hurt us, and the lack of support and the lack of community and the invisibility of illness, people's quickness to forget, their easy slip into denial. I have to walk and sing and write and plan for a future where we'll be able to do the things we want to do, despite everything, and to work as hard as possible to reach those goals. We were always big dreamers, and even scaled back dreams are more than most people think possible.

I think one of the biggest problems I had, and it's a problem I see a lot particularly in punk/activist circles, is I survived on crisis all my life. I didn't know how to slow down or sit with my feelings. But in order to be a good friend to this person I loved, and in order to be able to be who I wanted to be, I eventually I had to learn to stop running. At one point, I had repeated the same mistakes so many times that I had to make change a priority in my life. I had to learn to be still and present. I had to quit drinking. I had to look at the way I deal with stress and sadness and fear, and I had to feel it, process it, learn new ways of coping and living. I had to learn to be grounded and in my body. I'm still learning, and it's hard, but it's making everything much better, and I can actually do more and do it in more sustainable ways if I'm not doing it all out of panic, guilt or fear.

Noemi Martinez

trying to tell the truth

try to tell the truth
of weak legs that don't support
the heaviness of your heart
& all you want is that hand
supporting the arch in your back,
even in pain there is hope

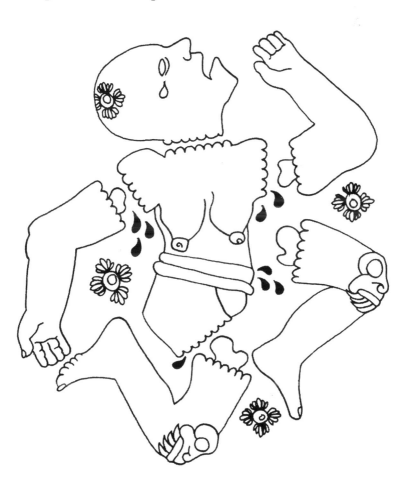

Karen Hixson & Jenna Goldin
with claire barrera & Meredith Butner

communication and supporting each other when facing chronic pain or illness

The following is text of a handout created for a reading and discussion event planned around the release of the first issue of the zine *When Language Runs Dry.*

It can be really difficult to communicate with each other about issues of chronic pain/illness. We live in a culture that perpetuates isolation by encouraging us not to let anyone see our pain and pressures us to take care of ourselves. But we need each other's support along the path of chronic pain/illness. No one can do it alone. While we might not always feel able to provide or ask for support due to our own limitations, it can be helpful for us to think ahead about our challenges and the type of support we'd like to provide to each other. When the opportunity to share moments of support comes up, we'll be more prepared to be there for each other. We've gathered some suggestions and ideas that we hope will be helpful but may not fit for everyone in all situations. Use your best judgment and intuition about what is needed.

BE PRESENT + VALIDATE

If someone gets vulnerable with you about their pain/illness or a loved one's current pain/illness/treatment/support needs, try to be present. Listen to them. Practice mindful listening without a need to do anything. Acknowledge and validate their experience with your own authentic words and body language. Be yourself. You don't have to be perfect. You don't have to have experienced something to validate it. ("That sounds really scary; I'm sorry it's been real hard lately; It makes sense you haven't been able to participate in X group/event.")

WATCH FOR PROBLEM SOLVING

Be aware about making suggestions or problem solving with the person. Is this what they have asked for? Is this a way to disconnect from more vulnerable emotions in the moment? Are you putting yourself in an expert, power-over role? Be careful of judgment around people's decisions on what medical care or lifestyle changes to pursue. Maintain your support despite them not taking the course of care you would recommend. Remember that many things could be impacting these decisions including, personal beliefs, financial restrictions or being overwhelmed. Meet someone where they're at. Even if it seems they are neglecting themselves, there is a context to each person's decisions.

REFLECT ON THE DIFFICULT MOMENTS + TALK ABOUT IT

Notice any discomfort or awkwardness in your communication or relationship, which could lead to pulling away from the moment or the person. These difficulties can lead to more chronic distance in otherwise close friendships. Try to share these feelings with the person if possible. Be vulnerable, especially if this is someone you have a relationship with who will allow you some room to be uncertain. ("I feel scared that you are feeling so bad; I'm worried I'm going to say the wrong thing right now; I don't know how to help." "I'm having a really hard time asking for help, so I am avoiding you." "I'm avoiding talking about things because I am scared to see you sad.") Many things get in the way of asking for and providing solid support including fear of saying the wrong thing or not knowing what to say. Some people may feel guilty that they are doing well, feeling good and are able-bodied.

Sometimes we need space to figure out what was making the moment difficult for us. Take some time to explore what was going on for you. Talk to another trusted person about it if you don't feel clear on what was happening. Go back to the person after thinking about the interaction and share your emotions, thoughts and reflections. ("I didn't realize I was being so distant when your talked with me yesterday; Thanks for talking with me about how you are doing; I realized that when you talk about your pain, it just makes me feel hopeless about mine. I don't want us to pull away from each other, what can we do?")

OFFER HELP + ATTEMPT TO PROVIDE SUSTAINABLE SUPPORT

Research your loved one's condition to have better understanding. Create space for someone to share what they feel/need instead of waiting for them to bring it up. While it is an individual's responsibility to ask for what they need, this can be really hard because of how we were raised and/or experiences we've had in like asking for and being denied what we need. Offering specific help like "Would it help if I went to the doctor with you?" or open-ended questions like "I really want to support you. What can I do to be helpful right now?" creates instant space for the person to share. Also be aware that some people aren't ready or comfortable accepting help yet, or maybe they can accept help but aren't yet able to process openly about the care giving relationship or about very vulnerable aspects of their situation/feelings. Accept people where they are. Obtain support and care from your own support system to avoid burnout as a caregiver.

TOLERATE DIFFICULT EMOTIONS

Notice that folks may feel more than one way about things or may have ambivalence about their situation. ("Sounds like sometimes you feel motivated and other times you want to give up on even trying.") Dark thoughts are not uncommon for folks dealing with chronic pain/illness. While these may be uncomfortable to hear, work on maintaining calm. Often people are not really suicidal but may just not want to be alive because they are in so much physical or emotional pain. People need to have the space for these feelings without their support system freaking out or misunderstanding.

There are ways to assess someone's suicidal risk without being immediately alarmed. Ask and assess:

- Sometimes when people feel sad, they have thoughts of harming or killing themselves. Have you been thinking about this seriously?
- Do you know how you would do it?
- Do you have the stuff around?
- I care about you and want you to be safe. Let's figure out a plan to make that happen.

As someone with chronic pain/illness:

Do your best to talk to someone you trust, seek supportive counseling with an educated and non-judgmental professional, don't stay in unhelpful counseling, read supportive materials not just about the content of your pain/illness but about how to deal with it emotionally. When ready, attempt to explore new, untapped parts of yourself that allow you to feel more alive, competent and connected.

CONSIDER THE CONTEXT OF THE PERSON'S LIFE

Attempt to consider and be aware of how class, race, gender, family history and all aspects of a person's identity play out in health related issues. Be aware when giving support/suggestions that not everyone has access to resources or can make the same lifestyle changes available to someone with more access to resources and support can.

In closing: let's not wait until one of these issues comes up to begin prioritizing them in our communities.

We would like to extend a special thanks to BEN HOLTZMAN for his article, "Illness and Support" which provided significant inspiration for this handout. You can read this article alongside many other important stories and essays about physical illness in the zine *Sick: a Compilation Zine on Physical Illness.*

Mobilization of Care & Support Through Communication

Stress, burnout and everyday trauma are influenced and maintained by disconnection and isolation. Self-blame, pressure, comparison, as well as our own desires to be more active, engaged and productive lead to states of immobilization. We are afraid to share what is happening with us. We fear burdening friends and family. We fear being judged. We fear speaking our full truth. We fear other people will blame themselves for our pain. We don't want to admit we struggle as we live in a society that values productivity, product and ability. It makes sense that we often don't know how or have difficulty finding the words or actions that will allow us to mobilize support. And, perhaps part of this burden of mobilizing support could be placed on our support system, neighbors, co-workers, etc., as they may be able to step up and support us in securing support when they see struggle, pain or disconnection within us or in our lives. Whether it is stress/anxiety/burnout or another issue including chronic pain, illness, mental health or relationship difficulties. We want to support people in conveying their difficulties to decrease isolation, disconnection and foster a sense of autonomy, empowerment and connection within our support systems and begin to create radical communities of care. These radical communities of care will begin with addressing the hard moments, the vulnerable moments, the challenging moments.

Questions to consider in mobilizing support:

1. What is one thing you wish you could tell a friend, family member, caregiver, partner, co-worker, supervisor, fellow activist or parent about something you are dealing with?

_____

_____

_____

_____

2. What would it take to feel comfortable doing so?

_____

_____

_____

_____

3. What are the words that would help you convey this?

_____

_____

_____

_____

4. What is the medium that is best for you? Face-to-face conversation, phone, email, letter or through another support person?

_____

_____

_____

_____

5. Are you willing to take the risk? If so, when?

_____

_____

_____

_____

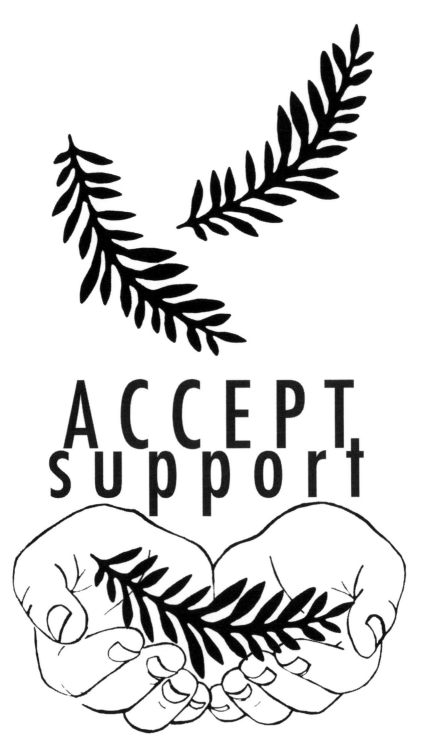

ACCEPT
support

further reading

About my Disappearance
Dave Roche
> Dave has made four honest, funny and heartbreaking issues of this zine about life with Crohn's disease. Search them out! (MB)

Acceptance And Commitment Therapy For Chronic Pain
Joanne Dahl, Kelly G. Wilson, Carmen Luciano, Steven C. Hayes

ADAPT
adapt.org

Aftershock: Confronting Trauma in a Violent World: A Guide for Activists and Their Allies
Pattrice Jones

The Alchemy of Illness
Kat Duff

The Body Keeps the Score: Brain, Mind, and Body in the Healing of Trauma
Bessel van der Kolk

The Body in Pain
Elaine Scarry

The Body is Not an Apology
thebodyisnotanapology.com

Breaking the Vicious Cycle: Intestinal Health Through Diet
Elaine Gottschall
> I found this book just after I finished drawing SICK. It talks about the connection between your brain and your guts, and the correlation between things like Crohn's, IBS, colitis, panic disorder, schizophrenia and autism. (AM)

Brown Star Girl
brownstargirl.org

This Bridge We Call Home: Radical Visions of Transformation
Gloria Anzaldua

The Chronic Pain Care Workbook: A Self-Treatment Approach to Pain Relief Using the Behavioral Assessment of Pain Questionnaire
Michael Lewandowski

> This workbook, developed by the psychologist responsible for the Behavioral Assessment of Pain Questionnaire used in pain centers worldwide, asks a series of questions designed to help a person experiencing chronic pain make sense of what they are facing physically and emotionally. Though I didn't complete every aspect of this workbook, I feel it was very useful in helping me find language to communicate my pain levels to doctors. Rating my answers to each question showed the varying types of emotional stresses that result from and contribute to my specific pain experience. This book provides tools for relaxation, healing, and self-care around the subjects that are individually the most challenging and problematic for each reader in particular. (MB)

Communities of Care, Organizations for Liberation
Yashna Maya Padamsee

> Essay can be found here: nayamaya.wordpress.com (KH)

Cutting Glass: A Zine About Vulvodynia

Creative Stress: A Path for Evolving Souls Living through Personal and Planetary Upheaval
James O'Dea

Crip Theory
Robert McRuer

The Culture of Pain
David Morris

> This book looks toward literature, history, art, psychology and medicine in an exploration of how modern society can attempt to make sense of and cope with the mystery of Chronic Pain. (MB)

Egoscue: Pain Free Workout

> I bought this DVD workout set after my uncle introduced me to some Egoscue method stretches and have felt a real benefit from following it. I'm still on the beginner disc - 40 minutes of low impact exercises focusing on posture, alignment and flexibility. (MB)

Explain Pain
David Butler
> Modern pain science and research explained in non-technical language. (MB)

Feminist Theory: From Margin to Center
bell hooks

Fibromyaligia and Chronic Myofascial Pain: A Survival Manual
Devyn Starlanyl

Freedom from Pain
Peter A. Levine

Harm Reduction Guide to Getting Off Psychiatric Drugs
The Icarus Project and Freedom Center
> This zine has lots of great information gleaned from other important sources, condensed into a little packet - with pictures. (AM)

Help for the Helper: The Psychophysiology of Compassion Fatigue and Vicarious Trauma
Babette Rothschild

Illness as Metaphor
Susan Sontag

The Language of Pain: Finding Words, Compassion, and Relief
David Biro
> A beautiful book about the power of metaphor to transform and communicate the pain experience. (MB)

Leaving Evidence
Leavingevidence.wordpress.com

Living Beyond Your Pain: Using Acceptance and Commitment Therapy to Ease Chronic Pain
Joanne Dahl + Tobias Lundgren

Loving in the War Years
Cherie Moraga

Mama Sick
mamasick.com
> Mama Sick is a blog by a mama with chronic illness. (CB)

Nobody Passes
nobodypasses.blogspot.com
> This is the blog of Mattilda Bernstein Sycamore, who also wrote the book So Many Ways to Sleep Badly. Sycamore is an awesome queer lady who has fibromyalgia which she often blogs about and relates to other issues in her life including queer/trans identity, abuse history, radical politics, etc. (CB)

It's Not the End of the World: Building a Life with Limp Wrists
Ocean Capewell
> In hand and wrist pain and fed up with the search to find books and materials about the condition as it related to life as a punk kid, zinester and dishwasher, Ocean put together this zine as a resource for other folks in pain. A great zine "full of occupation-specific hazards, and suggested remedies to help manage these hazards." Chock full of general advice, along with specific sections on bike delivery, dishwashing, construction, zine making, and cashiering to complete this "zine about carpal tunnel, tendonitis, and how to keep yr. job from ruining yr. life." (MB)

The Rejected Body: Feminist Philosophical Reflections on Disability
Susan Wendell

Sick: A Compilation Zine on Physical Illness
Ben Holtzman

Sins Invalid
sinsinvalid.org

Stitches: A Memoir
David Small
> This is my new favorite comic. It is amazing - read it. (AM)

Translucent Transformation: Interviews and Stories of Bodily Experiences
Christa Donner

I stumbled across visual artist Christa Donner's amazing work on the internet and ordered several of her health centered zines and brochures. She works with interview and personal narrative to bring together diverse perspectives. (MB)

Trauma Stewardship: An Everyday Guide to Caring for Self While Caring for Others
Laura van Dernoot Lipsky + Connie Burk

Under the Medical Gaze: Facts and Fictions about Chronic Pain
Susan Greenhaigh

What is Found There: Notebooks on Poetry and Politics
Adrienne Rich

I came back to this book during my injury because of Rich's passionate and powerful stance on the necessity of poetry as a tool for personal and political change. In a question central to the book, Rich asks writers to ask themselves "how to bear witness to a reality from which the public - and maybe part of the poet - wants, or is persuaded it wants, to turn away." When words fail me this collection of essays, lectures, notebook fragments and Rich's personal letters is always one to turn to for thoughtful, lyrical, and challenging thoughts about why language is important. (MB)

Woman Who Glows in the Dark
Elena Avila

This book is both an explanation of Curanderismo (the Mexican tradition of folk healing) and a memoir of Avila's journey to become a curandera - a holistic and powerful way of looking at health and healing. (CB)

The Woman Who Watches Over the World
Linda Hogan

Women's Bodies, Women's Wisdom: Creating Physical and Emotional Health and Healing
Christane Northrup

A good health resource in general, and it helped me understand both the personal and external causes of the physical and emotional ailments that affect women's lives. It's really validating, and caused me to view my own health in a more holistic, empowering way. (EK)

contributors

HEATHER ANDERSON found her heart in Oakland, her voice in Portland, and her brain in New York City. She recently moved to Los Angeles and endeavors to use her heart, voice and brain to support equity in the built environment. Heather continues with her love of walking, biking, drawing with pen, pencil or shitty xeroxes, and listening. If you are interested in contacting Heather, email her at: h.nicole.a@gmail.com

CLAIRE BARRERA is a mamma, dancer, writer and activist living in Portland, Oregon.

AJA ROSE BOND is an artist and community organizer with a background in music, craft and fashion respectively; drawing from the deep influence of D.I.Y. punk, queer feminisms and magic. Her past collaborative projects include the STAG Library, WOEVAN (Witches of East Vancouver), Her Jazz Noise Collective and Seamrippers Craft Collective. In 2014 she started the Witches* Union Hall which produced a collectively created, in-depth zine and workshop on Cultural Appropriation in Spirituality. Most recently she has been working on a personal, comic-style zine called Home Body, about magic, politics and healing. ajarosebond.com / witchesunionhall.wordpress.com / email: ajarosebond@gmail.com

MEREDITH BUTNER is a writer and painter living in Portland, Oregon. She answers most of the mail for this project: chronicpainzine@gmail.com

CINDY CRABB writes the long running, feminist/ autobiographical zine "Doris". She has also compiled and edited the zines "Support," "Learning Good Consent," "Filling the Void: interviews about quitting drinking and using," and "Masculinities." Visit her website: dorisdorisdoris.com, or write: pob 29 / Athens Ohio 45701

JONAH ALINE DANIEL is a gender variant, chronically ill, energetic herbalist, candle maker, organizer and descendent of Russian, Lithuanian, and English Jews. they are committed to racial and economic justice, disability and healing justice, radical liberatory earth based Judaism, environmental justice, and to a process of de-colonization, reparation, and repair. these days they are living rurally on Makahmo Southern Pomo land (also called north sonoma county, california) caring for chickens and bees and soo many medicinal plants, making plant medicine and beeswax Jewish ritual candles that support the full Palestinian call for Boycott of israeli goods. they love snail mail and planned visits!

900 Hiatt Rd Unit B
Cloverdale, CA 95425
jonahalinedaniel@gmail.com
www.narrowbridgecandles.org

KORI DOTY & ANDI GRACE: andi and Kori live on a quaint little queer and trans land project called 'the homostead' on un-ceded sinixt territory. andi is an author, herbalist, facilitator and all around kitchen witch. You can check out their work on their website: www.andigracewrites.com. Kori is an author, facilitator, maker and life coach. You can find their work at: www.koridoty.com.

SUNNY DRAKE is a femme, queer & trans writer, performer & educator. He's toured his award-winning theater shows extensively in Australia, the USA, Canada and Europe. He is also the author of a blog which weaves trans and queer politics with personal story (www.sunnydrake.com).

JENNA GOLDIN is a Licensed Tax Return Preparer in Portland, Oregon. She is a partner at Math LLC (mathllc.com), a tax preparation, consulting and bookkeeping business that focuses on small businesses and creatives. Her goal is to make accounting more accessible and empowering for all people.

ANNA HAMILTON (nom de web Annaham) is a government employee, chronically ill person, and disability rights advocate by day. A writer who has contributed articles, cartoons, and more to publications such as xoJane, Bitch Magazine, The Toast, and Global Comment, she is also the Managing Editor of Disability Intersections. She lives near Sacramento, California, and enjoys writing humorous personal essays (all stuck in various stages of revision), spending time with her partner and their aging Yorkie, and experimenting with weird eye makeup looks. You can contact her by visiting her website at: annaham.net, or email her: hamdotblog@gmail.com.

KAREN HIXSON is a counselor, educator and supervisor in Portland, Oregon. She works to create supportive, engaging and authentic therapeutic relationships that value the cultural context. Karen is currently working on her dissertation entitled Understanding Power in Therapeutic Relationships. She can be reached at karenhixson@mac.com

SAILOR HOLLADAY is a writer, textile artist, and asset builder with low income communities across Oregon. www.sailorholladay.com

CRAIG-JESSE HUGHES lives in New York City. He is a member of the Team Colors Collective and works as a social worker in harm reduction services. He can be reached at craig@warmachines.info.

MEADOW JONES is a feminist writer, new media artist and educator living in Urbana Illinois. All of her work returns to the same open inquiries, what are the points of intervention in systems of violence, and how do we make the world we want to live in.

EMILY KLAMER lives in St. Louis, Missouri, where she is a graduate student in Clinical Mental Health Counseling. Emily is particularly interested in examining the intersections of trauma and social justice, and is engaged in community advocacy work to raise awareness regarding toxic stress and personal and collective trauma. In her spare time, Emily can be found trying to catch up on her New Yorker subscription and cuddling with her cat, Ruby.

CRAIG LEWIS a Psychiatric Survivor, Mental Health Expert by Experience, author, lifelong punk rocker, activist, anti-authoritarian, cat-lover, workshop trainer, international speaker, and much more. Craig has survived a lifetime of struggle and has chosen to not allow his suffering to be wasted. Craig shares of his experiences, knowledge and lessons learned, in hopes of supporting others in living happier, healthier and more satisfying lives. This is an ongoing journey and Craig, like all of us, is a work in progress. Craig has authored Better Days - A Mental Health Recovery Workbook - WWW.BETTERDAYSRECOVERY.COM - and compiled and published 'You're Crazy - Volume One', the first in a series of first-hand accounts of people from the punk scene who deal with mental health struggle, addiction and trauma - WWW.PUNKSINRECOVERY.COM - Craig lives in Salem, MA with his best four legged twenty-eight toed friend, Max the Cat. Craig no longer identifies as having a "mental illness" and is now aware that he never had the alleged symptoms for which he was labeled as "mentally ill" for and then manipulatively and fraudulently treated for. Craig is now free of all psychiatric medications and he is focused on living the healthiest, happiest and most satisfying life possible, while doing all that he can to help nurture and facilitate the same for others. Craig is open to any and all communication and people can email him at: betterdaysrecovery@gmail.com

NOEMI MARTINEZ is a poet, community worker, sociocultural critic and full time bruja living in South Texas. While living through chronic illness Noemi also earned a master's in history and writing, sat by her daughter's side as she was in a coma from an acquired brain injury and wrote lines of poems and medical words on slips of paper. She still prefers playing with oil pastels, gesso and creating erasure poetry.

MELANNIE MCKENZIE is a poet and multi-disciplinary artist and educator utilizing text, textiles, performance art and digital media to explore themes of grief, trauma, resilience, and intersectionality. as a queer, chronically ill & disabled, black-taino artist, melannie is ardent about interdependence, the pursuit of justice and in presenting the union of art and activism as agents of change in our present and future realities. among their goals are: learn to swim, write a book(s), and dismantle all systems of oppression. melannie is, as always, a work in progress.

ANNIE MURPHY I am a Portland-born writer and drawer committed to figuring out what's going on inside my body, mind, spirit, world. I self-published the zines Fear of Fear - a Journal of Psychological Resistance, and Witch Hunt: Addressing Mental Health and Confronting Sexual Assault in Activist Communities, drew a suit for the Collective Tarot, and received a Xeric grant for my comic I Still Live: Biography of a Spiritualist. I also edited the Ignatz Award-nominated Gay Genius comics anthology. If you wanna talk about my stuff, my email's murphylawless@gmail.com. Or if you like comics, go to ghostcatcomics.blogspot.com.

CASSANDRA J. PERRY is a narcoleptic insomniac and a hypermobile gimp, among other diagnoses. She is studying the intersection of chronic pain with sadomasochism, and more generally disability and sexuality. Using a variety of monikers and platforms, Cassandra has written publicly and extensively on issues of sex, relationships, disability, and mental health since before she was old enough to know better. She is devoted to her two cats and her pseudo-kiddo. She can be found at cassandrajperry.com.

MARISSA RAGUET currently lives in the Twin Cities where she works in the field of sexual violence prevention. Feel free to contact: mjoy49@gmail.com

NITIKA RAJ is a spiritual revolutionary and glorious femme. After working in anti-violence, racial justice, and economic justice movements for 12 years, she founded Moksh Creative Consulting through which she offers organizational consulting and professional coaching services. She is also a passionate board member of the Astraea Lesbian Foundation for Justice. In 2015, Nitika co-produced, co-directed and performed in Yoni ki Raat (Night of Vagina), a theater production to raise awareness about issues of gender, sexuality, and violence in the South Asian community. Her writing has been published in Tikkun magazine (2013), Criptiques: an anthology of writing on disability (2014), Anti-Oppressive Social Work Practice (2014), Queering Sexual Violence (2016), and various online forums. Nitika has also edited and produced two zines for social justice organizations - 33 Cups of Chai (for Chaya in 2010), and To the Left and Write (for Western States Center in 2010). Born in India and raised in Kuwait, she currently lives in and loves from New York City. You can reach her at nitika.raj@gmail.com.

ELIZABETH ROBERTSON lives in Portland, Oregon, where

she goes to medical appointments like it's her job and attempts to knit the pain away at home. She is a queer, femme, magical creature committed to destroying the white supremacist-capitalist-heteronormative-patriarchy through beauty, creativity, defense of the wild, and diversity of tactics. She can be reached for art and ideas at elizuhbethr@gmail.com

HENRY RODRIGUEZ for more artwork by Henry Rodriguez visit: www.tattoosbyhenry.com

E.T. RUSSIAN is an artist, author, filmmaker, performer, educator and healthcare provider living in Seattle, Washington. Russian is the author of The Ring of Fire Anthology (2014) and has published work in The Graphic Medicine Manifesto (2015), Gay Genius (2011) and The Collective Tarot (2008). Russian is a current member of Seattle comic collective THE HAND, co-founded the Seattle Disability Justice Collective (2012), has performed in productions by Sins Invalid and dance company Light Motion, and co-directed the movie Third Antenna: A documentary about the radical nature of drag (2001). Russian has lectured at Universities, conferences and community organizations across the country, and received grant support from The Art Matters Foundation (2014) and the Harlan Hahn Award in Disability Studies from the University of Washington (2013, 2015). Russian is a documentarian at heart and believes storytelling is a powerful tool for the liberation of all people. Learn more at ETRUSSIAN.COM

SHELBY graduated Summa Cum Laude from the Maryland Institute College of Art with a degree in Printmaking, Book Arts and Art History in May 2014. Since then she has worked at Johns Hopkins University's Milton S. Eisenhower Library as a Conservation Technician, and is currently finishing a research appointment exploring the potential of incorporating 3D printing technologies into a library environment. She will be applying for a Masters in Library Science and Information Systems this spring. When she isn't working at the library she's slinging coffee drinks as a barista, and wishing she was home cooking Cuban cuisine with her cat.

STARLING is a thinker by nurture, and a mystic and creator by nature. While originally from London England, she now lives in so called Montreal where she is learning about the possibilities of healing and living in the presence of toxicity and contradictions. She is nourished by working with the Mad Pride 'Montreal' collective and the Work that Reconnects. She feels freer than ever when she sings, especially in places of passage like streets, the subway, and on trains.

CORINNE TEED's work broadly explores marginalized identities in the context of human and non-human interactions, often focusing on queer relationality, cross species empathy and the poetics of ecological thought. In her work, Corinne utilizes printmaking, drawing, installation, time-based media and participatory practices. Corinne received a BA from Brown University and an MFA at the University or Iowa. www.corinneteed.net

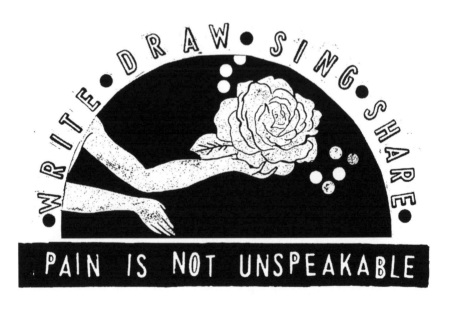

Printed in Great Britain
by Amazon

36285319R00126